100 Questions & Answers About Gastrointestinal Stromal Tumor (GIST)

Ronald P. DeMatteo, MD

Hepatobiliary Service
Memorial Sloan-Kettering Cancer Center
New York, NY

Marina Symcox, PhD

GIST Support International
Bristow, OK

George D. Demetri, MD

Sarcoma Center
Dana-Farber Cancer Institute
Boston, MA

JONES AND BARTLETT PUBLISHERS
Sudbury, Massachusetts
BOSTON   TORONTO   LONDON   SINGAPORE

World Headquarters
Jones and Bartlett Publishers
40 Tall Pine Drive
Sudbury, MA 01776
978-443-5000
info@jbpub.com
www.jbpub.com

Jones and Bartlett Publishers
Canada
6339 Ormindale Way
Mississauga, Ontario L5V 1J2
CANADA

Jones and Bartlett Publishers
International
Barb House, Barb Mews
London W6 7PA
UK

Jones and Bartlett's books and products are available through most bookstores and online booksellers. To contact Jones and Bartlett Publishers directly, call 800-832-0034, fax 978-443-8000, or visit our website, www.jbpub.com.

Substantial discounts on bulk quantities of Jones and Bartlett's publications are available to corporations, professional associations, and other qualified organizations. For details and specific discount information, contact the special sales department at Jones and Bartlett via the above contact information or send an email to specialsales@jbpub.com.

Production Credits
Executive Publisher: Christopher Davis
Editorial Assistant: Kathy Richardson
Production Director: Amy Rose
Associate Production Editor: Daniel Stone
Marketing Associate: Laura Kavigian

Manufacturing and Inventory Coordinator:
  Therese Connell
Composition: Appingo
Cover Design: Kate Ternullo
Cover Image: © Photodisc
Printing and Binding: Malloy, Inc.
Cover Printing: Malloy, Inc.

Library of Congress Cataloging-in-Publication Data
DeMatteo, Ronald.
   100 Q&A about gastrointestinal stromal tumors (GIST) / Ronald DeMatteo, George D. Demetri, Marina Symcox.
      p. cm.
   ISBN-13: 978-0-7637-3838-9
   ISBN-10: 0-7637-3838-7
   1. Gastrointestinal stromal tumors—Miscellanea. 2. Gastrointestinal stromal tumors—Popular works. I. Demetri, George D., 1956– II. Symcox, Marina. III. Title. IV. Title: One hundred Q&A about gastrointestinal stromal tumors (GIST). V. Title: 100 Q and A about gastrointestinal stromal tumors (GIST). VI. Title: 100 questions & answers about gastrointestinal stromal tumors (GIST).
   RC280.D5D46 2007
   616.3'3—dc22
                                        2006031327
6048

The authors, editor, and publisher have made every effort to provide accurate information. However, they are not responsible for errors, omissions, or for any outcomes related to the use of the contents of this book and take no responsibility for the use of the products and procedures described. Treatments and side effects described in this book may not be applicable to all people; likewise, some people may require a dose or experience a side effect that is not described herein. Drugs and medical devices are discussed that may have limited availability controlled by the Food and Drug Administration (FDA) for use only in a research study or clinical trial. Research, clinical practice, and government regulations often change the accepted standard in this field. When consideration is being given to use of any drug in the clinical setting, the health care provider or reader is responsible for determining FDA status of the drug, reading the package insert, and reviewing prescribing information for the most up-to-date recommendations on dose, precautions, and contraindications, and determining the appropriate usage for the product. This is especially important in the case of drugs that are new or seldom used.

Printed in the United States of America
10 09 08 07   10 9 8 7 6 5 4 3 2 1

CONTENTS

Contents

Gastrointestinal stromal tumor (GIST) has emerged in recent years as one of the most tremendous success stories in cancer research and therapy. While GIST is an uncommon cancer, it has unique properties making it a model for a new frontier in cancer medicine called "targeted cancer therapy." These days, patients whose GIST cannot be surgically cured are enjoying dramatically better chances of survival and control of their disease due to new breakthrough drugs. In addition to being far more effective than older forms of cancer therapy (chemotherapy), these new drugs have important practical benefits: they can be taken by patients at home as oral pills or capsules, and they are reasonably well tolerated so that patients can enjoy acceptable quality of life over the course of years of continuous treatment. The revolutionary advancements in the care of GIST patients are quite remarkable when we consider that even less than ten years ago, doctors lacked reliable methods to accurately diagnosis GIST, and worse yet, there was nothing at all in the arsenal of standard anti-cancer therapies that could treat GIST effectively. But with the arrival of imatinib in the first clinical trials for GIST in the year 2000 as the first targeted cancer therapy, and the introduction of sunitinib in 2002 as a second option for GIST patients if imatinib fails, the outlook for GIST patients has improved dramatically. This once "orphan disease" and overlooked cancer has gained wide recognition in recent years as the topic of plenary lectures at professional oncology conferences and as the subject of medical news stories in the popular news media.

A new GIST diagnosis brings to patients and their families not only many personal adjustments, but also the challenges of learning new medical concepts and making decisions about the best medical care. Patients and families want to retain some measure of control over their own situation and be their own advocates in the health care system. Gathering practical information and knowing enough to ask the right questions of your doctor and health care team are both aspects of dealing with cancer. We wrote *100 Questions & Answers About Gastrointestinal Stromal Tumor (GIST)* to give our readers an overview of the major and sometimes novel concepts that have become very relevant to GIST patients in recent years. We have tried to provide simple yet accurate explanations about the biology of GIST and how targeted cancer therapies block the major defects that are responsible for the cancerous behavior of GIST cells. The advent of targeted therapies for GIST in recent years has also brought a new set of considerations for doctors and patients regarding the optimal way to manage the disease and how to evaluate the clinical response of GIST to these drugs. We appreciate that a GIST diagnosis brings many new psychological, social, and working concerns to a family's daily routine. We share with you some of the emotional insights and practical tips that might help you and your friends and relatives cope better with your diagnosis.

So what are important things for a newly diagnosed GIST patient to keep in mind? First, many patients with early GIST that is limited to one part of the body may still be cured by expert surgery alone. However, even when surgeons cannot cure a patient with more advanced GIST, this disease is now manageable as a long-term, chronic condition for many patients. GIST patients are able to lead fairly normal lives with only mild side effects from their targeted cancer therapy. Still we should point out that GIST remains a serious and potentially life threatening disease. Patients diagnosed with GIST need to be committed to take their oral cancer drugs, and to be vigilant about having routine medical check ups for many years to come.

The authors of this book represent the combined voices of a surgical oncologist, a GIST patient, and a medical oncologist. In addition, a registered nurse provided editorial guidance and additional material for this volume. Each of us brings to this project a unique perspective as either a health care professional or a GIST patient.

The Surgeon's Journey with GIST before and after Imatinib

Ronald DeMatteo, MD, became interested in GIST in 1998 because of the lack of effective therapies for it. In fact, surgery was used quite commonly at that time for patients with metastatic GIST since conventional chemotherapy was essentially ineffective. While he and his colleagues were trying to develop a new approach using intraperitoneal chemotherapy for metastatic GIST, it became clear that a new agent then known as "STI571" (now called imatinib mesylate) was efficacious. Dr. DeMatteo went on to lead 2 national clinical trials of adjuvant imatinib after the resection of primary GIST. These trials are sponsored by the National Cancer Institute and Novartis Pharmaceuticals and are being led by the American College of Surgeons Oncology Group. He, along with a team of investigators at Memorial Sloan-Kettering Cancer Center, have contributed to our current understanding of the clinical management of patients with primary or metastatic GIST and the mechanism of imatinib resistance.

The Patient's Journey with GIST before and after Imatinib

Marina Symcox, PhD, is a retired biochemist who was diagnosed at age 38 years with advanced terminal GIST in 1997. She fought a losing battle against GIST in the era of the late 1990's before the arrival of effective therapies. At one point she spent eight months in hospice and came close to death. In 2000, she became one of the first patients in the world to receive imatinib as an experimental drug. Continuing with six years of successful imatinib therapy, she has recovered to lead a normal and active life. In the nine years since her diagnosis, Marina has been an active member of Internet support groups for patients. Marina has brought to *100 Questions & Answers About Gastrointestinal Stromal Tumor (GIST)* her insights regarding what patients on the Internet would like to know about GIST biology, treatments, and coping in the face of terminal disease.

The Medical Oncologist's Journey with GIST before and after Imatinib

George Demetri, MD, has spent the majority of his professional career developing new drugs against solid tumors such as GIST and other sarcomas. Working with a network of colleagues across the world, Dr. Demetri's team was the first to give imatinib to patients with GIST, and later followed similar scientific paths to successfully treat imatinib-resistant GIST patients with sunitinib. Dr. Demetri has brought together a coalition of investigators and universities globally with support from large pharmaceutical firms including Novartis and Pfizer, smaller biotechnology firms such as Sugen and Infinity, as well as the U.S. National Cancer Institute and the philanthropic foundation of the Ludwig Trust for Cancer Research. The work from this team has formed the basis for the U.S. Food and Drug Administration (FDA) approval of imatinib and sunitinib as safe and effective therapies for GIST, and is also forming the foundation of future research to improve further the effectiveness of targeted cancer therapies.

We would like to extend a warm thank you to Chris Davis, Executive Publisher for the medical list at Jones and Bartlett Publishers, Inc. His unwavering encouragement for this project, from the time it was conceptualized 2 years ago, deserves recognition as the keystone between concept and implementation that has brought this book to GIST patients and their families.

Ronald P. DeMatteo, MD
Memorial Sloan-Kettering Cancer Center

Marina Symcox, PhD
GIST survivor, GIST Support International

George D. Demetri, MD
Sarcoma Center, Dana-Farber Cancer Institute, Boston

Karla Knight, RN
Healthcare writer

GIST and the Revolution of Mechanism–Directed "Targeted Cancer Therapy"

We would like to give a brief historical overview of how GIST and the emerging field of drug development specifically targeting the molecular mechanisms of cancer were brought together to establish a new paradigm for cancer treatment. We have learned from GIST that even the most difficult and aggressive cancers can respond well to anticancer drugs once we have uncovered the fundamental molecular abnormalities which drive the cancer cell and then design drugs rationally to block these abnormalities. In the past and even today, most cancers are treated by toxic chemotherapy drugs that kill cells through nonspecific actions that can also harm normal cells. For GIST, however, conventional forms of toxic chemotherapy were nearly always ineffective. The application of targeted cancer therapies to GIST has provided the "proof of concept" to validate a new approach in oncology.

As recently as the late 1990's, the disease we now know as GIST was an intractable problem in the oncology clinic and an enigma for cancer researchers. For a long time, GIST was not even recognized as a distinct disease although Drs. Mazur and Clark had introduced the term "stromal tumor" in 1983 to describe a subset of tumors from the muscular wall of the GI tract that did not fit well into the standard classifications of cancers arising from this anatomic site. GIST patients throughout the 1990's were frequently told that their disease was a variant of another known cancer, "gastrointestinal leiomyosarcoma" (a smooth muscle cancer). We can't really say that GIST patients during this time were misdiagnosed, since GIST as a whole was so poorly understood.

GIST stood out as a frustrating problem in the clinic because the disease in patients simply did not respond to any conventional chemotherapy drugs.

Surgery was the only option to help patients with these tumors. Because GIST often spreads aggressively to other locations in the body, surgery was not sufficient to stop the course of the disease for many patients. Prior to the year 2000, patients with advanced GIST that had spread beyond the original tumor generally died within 1-2 years.

A landmark research discovery reported in January 1998 set in motion a series of major events that would completely revolutionize cancer medicine. Furthermore, these events would become a paradigm for how other types of solid tumors might be treated in the future. A Japanese research team that included Hirota and Kitamura had noticed that these poorly understood tumors from the GI wall expressed a mutant form of a protein called "KIT." The *KIT* gene had been previously identified over a decade earlier by Peter Besmer of Sloan-Kettering Institute. Only a few types of normal cells appeared to rely upon the signals conveyed through this KIT protein. One of the normal cell types dependent upon KIT protein is a specialized class known as the interstitial cells of Cajal (ICC); these normal cells are found in the muscular wall of the GI tract and generate the slow wave contractions of the GI tract during digestion. Hirota and his team postulated that GIST originated from the ICCs or else their more primitive precursors (stem cells). This insight provided the needed rationale to fully classify GIST as an entirely distinct disease entity from smooth muscle tumors from the GI wall (leiomyosarcoma) in which GIST had once been sub-classified.

Most importantly, this Japanese team discovered that these abnormal versions of KIT protein sent powerful signals into the GIST cells for them to grow continuously and to evade cell death. The activity of this abnormal KIT protein itself appeared to explain the fact that conventional chemotherapy drugs of all kinds fail to treat GIST.

Other researchers in Oregon, such as Dr. Michael Heinrich, and Boston, including Drs. Jonathan Fletcher, David Tuveson, Brian Rubin, and others also recognized the potential to intervene therapeutically by interrupting the abnormal signals from the mutant KIT protein. Fortunately, the tools to intervene were being developed for completely different reasons, and teams worldwide were then able to quickly connect the discovery of the abnormal KIT protein in GIST to a new drug originally designed to treat a particular cancer of white blood cells. The drug imatinib was among the first of a class of drugs called targeted cancer therapy that stop cancer cells by a radically different way than conventional chemotherapy. "Smart" drugs or so-called "targeted therapy" hone into the exact molecular abnormalities within the cancer cells and shut them off. Imatinib was created as part of a project in the 1980's and early 1990's at the Swiss pharmaceutical company Ceiba-Geigy (now Novartis) that designed drugs to stop the activity of certain types of proteins. Though much less was known about cancer cells in those days, the leaders of this project hypothesized that a category of proteins called "protein kinases" might be important in causing cancer, and that drugs stopping these protein kinases might be effective therapies for cancer patients. (E. Buchdunger, J. Zimmerman, Alex Matter, Nick Lydon). Imatinib was initially designed as an inhibitor of the Platelet-Derived Growth Factor Receptor (PDGFR) with the aim of using this to help patients with hardening of the arteries (coronary atherosclerosis). Importantly, imatinib was also potent in its ability to shut off the signals from an abnormal signaling protein called bcr-abl. Abnormal bcr-abl causes the development of a blood cancer called chronic myelogenous leukemia (CML).

Dr. Brian Druker, a hematologist at Oregon Health Science University, pioneered important studies of imatinib for this leukemia in both a pre-clinical laboratory setting and later as an unprecedented breakthrough therapy for CML patients. Dr. Druker also determined another important aspect of imatinib: in addition to blocking the bcr-abl protein in CML, imatinib could also block the actions of the KIT protein. At the time, the action of imatinib to block KIT was considered to be an unintended secondary effect. Dr. Druker's observation about imatinib and KIT in the mid-1990's had no application to the leukemia he was studying. About five years would pass before this observation had an application for another disease, which came once it was realized that the cancerous behaviors of GIST were driven by an abnormal KIT protein.

Researchers in Boston subsequently demonstrated in 1999 that imatinib was highly effective at killing GIST cells grown in a laboratory dish, and the same phenomenon could be demonstrated in other forms of blood cancer with *KIT* mutations tested in Oregon. This was an exciting discovery since up until that point no other drugs had seemed to work to kill GIST cells. Imatinib's activity to shut off the mutant KIT protein was a serendipitous turn of fortune for a desperate population of GIST patients who up until this point had never had any effective drug therapies. In mid 2000, the first group of GIST patients began to take imatinib as an experimental drug in a small clinical study conducted at Dana Farber Cancer Institute, Fox Chase Cancer Center, Oregon Health Sciences University, and Helsinki Finland. The early results were nothing short of spectacular. Patients who had once been extremely ill or even near death with advanced GIST experienced significant reductions in their tumors from their imatinib treatments. These astonishing results proved a major concept beyond any doubt. The key to successfully stopping GIST tumors is to treat patients with drugs that shut off the abnormal KIT protein harbored within them. Imatinib was quickly tested in hundreds more GIST patients and approved by the United States Food and Drug Administration (FDA) in 2002 as a breakthrough drug to treat GIST, quickly following on the FDA approval of imatinib as a safe and effective drug to treat CML patients.

Today—six years later—some of the GIST patients who first received imatinib as an experimental therapy continue to do very well. They report nearly normal lives despite the fact that they once had suffered from advanced GIST disease. In 2006, GIST came to the research headlines for a second time as treatable by another new oral cancer drug that was designed to inhibit multiple molecular targets in tumors: both by inhibiting the signaling through KIT and by stopping the formation of new blood vessels to feed the tumors. This new drug is called sunitinib. Drugs that interfere with the ability of cancerous tumors to recruit new blood vessels are called anti-angiogenesis agents. It was postulated as early as 1971 by Dr. Judah Folkman in Boston and Professor Robert Kerbel in Toronto, Canada, that such drugs might be able to prevent cancers from growing larger while having less toxic adverse side effects for patients. With sunitinib, GIST has again emerged as a model system at the frontier of testing another important paradigm, in this case multi-targeting of mutant enzyme signaling as well as inhibition of tumor-driven angiogenesis. This approach will likely be expanded to be tested in many other types of cancer, so the knowledge gained from GIST will impact upon the lives of many thousands of other cancer patients worldwide.

For now and into the future, the "holy grail" of cancer research is to uncover the exact nature of the molecular and genetic defects driving a cancer cell and then to match these against targeted cancer therapies designed to stop them. As a genetically simple type of solid tumor with seemingly straight-forward defects in a limited number of key pathways, GIST continues to be a research model of fundamental importance for unraveling what has gone wrong in a cancer cell at the molecular level. In a remarkably short period of six years, GIST has become a high-priority subject of clinical trials that test new experimental drugs. Patients with drug-resistant forms of GIST will no doubt benefit eventually from this research. Additionally, although breakthrough drugs such as imatinib and sunitinib have important clinical benefits for GIST patients when used individually, curative cancer therapy rarely, if ever, relies on a single drug. Almost certainly, combinations of drugs aimed at normalizing several key pathways in cancer cells will be required to move forward the next step. From the lessons learned from the biology and treatment of GIST, we can now rationally envision a future era of personalized cancer medicine targeted and customized to match a patient's own individually-unique spectrum of cancer cell defects.

Marina Symcox, PhD
GIST survivor, GIST Support International

Ronald P. DeMatteo, MD
Memorial Sloan-Kettering Cancer Center

George D. Demetri, MD
Sarcoma Center, Dana-Farber Cancer Institute, Boston

PART ONE

The Basics

What are the anatomy and function of the
gastrointestinal tract?

What is a gastrointestinal stromal tumor?

How are GISTs different than common cancers
of the stomach and intestines?

More . . .

1. What are the anatomy and function of gastrointestinal tract?

Gastrointestinal tract

The mouth, esophagus, stomach, small intestine, large intestine, rectum, and anus.

Esophagus

Primarily a passageway that pushes and moves food to the stomach.

Rectum

Approximately 12 cm long and functions as a storage tank of fecal material at the end of the large intestine; emptied on defecation.

Saliva

A substance in the mouth that provides lubrication and initiates digestion

Duodenum

First 12 inches of the small intestine.

Bile

A brownish, greenish fluid made in the liver and stored in the gallbladder; travels via the bile duct into the second portion of the duodenum. Bile helps in the digestion of fat.

The **gastrointestinal tract** includes the mouth, **esophagus**, stomach, small intestine, large intestine, **rectum**, and anus (Figure 1). Each portion of the gastrointestinal tract has a slightly different function. In the mouth, food is chewed, and **saliva** lubricates it and begins digestion. The esophagus is a passageway that pushes food to the stomach. The stomach resembles a washing machine as it churns food around to break it up even further. The small intestine is responsible for absorbing nutrients into the bloodstream. The first part is called the **duodenum**. **Bile** is made in the liver, is stored in the gallbladder, and travels via the bile duct into the second portion of the duodenum. Bile helps in the digestion of fat. Pancreatic juice also enters the duodenum and assists in

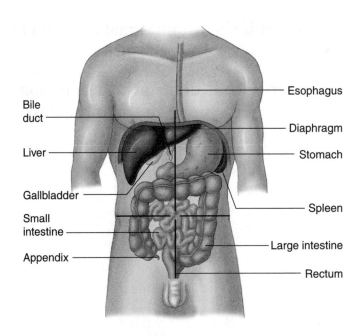

Bile duct
Liver
Gallbladder
Small intestine
Appendix

Esophagus
Diaphragm
Stomach
Spleen
Large intestine
Rectum

Figure 1   Gastrointestinal tract. The human GI tract includes the stomach, small intestine (made up of the duodenum, jejunum, and ileum), colon, and rectum.

protein and fat digestion. The large intestine (or **colon** as it is commonly called) reabsorbs water and salts from the intestinal contents. The rectum is a storage tank for fecal material that is cleared when your bowels are emptied.

2. What is a gastrointestinal stromal tumor?

A **gastrointestinal stromal tumor** (GIST) is a type of **cancer** known as **sarcoma**. Sarcomas are uncommon tumors, with about 8,000 to 10,000 new patients diagnosed every year in the United States. This is in contrast to lung cancer, prostate cancer, breast cancer, and colon cancer, each of which occurs in approximately 150,000 patients per year in this country. Sarcomas arise from components of nerve tissue, connective tissue, or muscle and therefore can occur anywhere in the body. A GIST is thought to originate from a special type of nerve cell in the gastrointestinal tract called the intestinal cell of Cajal. These cells normally function to regulate the contractions of the gastrointestinal tract during digestion.

The term GIST has only been widely used in the last 10 to 15 years. Before that, physicians thought that GISTs were actually **leiomyosarcomas**, another type of sarcoma that can arise from the gastrointestinal tract. GISTs are now clearly much more common than gastrointestinal leiomyosarcomas.

A GIST can occur anywhere in the gastrointestinal tract. A GIST most commonly (50% of the time) arises in the stomach, where it is called a stomach or gastric GIST. The next most frequent site is the small intestine. About 10% of the time, a GIST starts in the colon or the esophagus. Rarely (less than 5% of the time), a GIST originates within the abdomen but is not attached to the gastrointestinal tract.

A GIST has a very particular pattern of growth. Unlike most cancers, sarcomas tend to push surrounding structures instead of invading them. Nevertheless, by pushing on nearby organs, they may stick to them. One of the consequences of this is

Colon

Also called the large intestine; reabsorbs water and salts from the intestinal contents.

Gastrointestinal stromal tumor

A type of cancer classified as a sarcoma. GIST is thought to originate from a special type of nerve cell in the gastrointestinal tract called the intestinal cell of Cajal.

Cancer

A group of diseases in which cells grow abnormally.

Sarcomas

Cancers that arise from components of nerve tissue, connective tissue, or muscle and therefore can occur anywhere in the body.

Leiomyosarcomas

Another type of sarcoma that can arise from the gastrointestinal tract; less common than GISTs.

Adenocarcinoma

Cancer that begins in cells that line certain internal organs and that has glandular (secretory) properties; most cancers of the stomach and intestines are adenocarcinoma.

Epithelial cells

Cells that cover the surface of the body and line its cavities.

Lymphoma

Cancer that arises from cells in the immune system.

Neuroendocrine

Relating to the hormones of endocrine glands.

Cell

Smallest structural unit of an organism.

Primary site

The initial site of origin of a cancer.

Metastasis

The process of spreading cancer cells from the primary site to somewhere else in the body.

that sarcomas can become quite large before they produce symptoms. GISTs tend to grow off from a part of the gastrointestinal tract, somtimes with a stalk. Consequently, in many patients, only a small amount of normal tissue is taken to remove a GIST.

3. How are GISTs different than common cancers of the stomach and intestines?

Most other cancers of the gastrointestinal tract belong to a group of cancers called carcinomas or **adenocarcinomas**. **Adenocarcinomas** arise from **epithelial cells** that line the inside of the intestines. When patients are said to have a stomach or colon cancer, they usually have stomach or colon adenocarcinoma. Because a GIST is uncommon, patients with a GIST should be said to have a stomach or intestinal GIST. Of course, a variety of other tumors, such as **lymphoma** and **neuroendocrine** tumors, affect the stomach and intestines. Each type of cancer in the body has distinct features and behaves differently; thus, it is important to be specific.

4. What is cancer? What is the difference between a benign tumor and a malignant tumor?

Different components of the body, including the gastrointestinal tract, are made of **cells**—the smallest structural unit of a living organism. Normally, cells are born and die, and therefore, the body always needs new cells. This process is tightly regulated. Occasionally, a cell becomes capable of dividing in an uncontrolled fashion, leading to the formation of a tumor that contains abnormal cells.

The origin of a cancer is called the **primary site**. Thus, a primary gastric GIST began in the stomach. Cancer cells also have the ability to invade the bloodstream and spread to other sites within the body. This is called **metastasis**. A GIST that has spread to the liver is called a "GIST liver metastasis" or a "metastatic GIST involving the liver." At the time of diagnosis, one fourth of the patients have a primary GIST that has already metastasized. Physicians describe such a patient as having synchronous (i.e., at the same time) metastasis.

A **benign tumor** is abnormal tissue that may become a larger size. Unlike a cancer, however, a benign tumor does not spread to surrounding tissue or other organs. Some physicians describe certain GISTs as benign; however, "benign" can be very confusing and should generally be avoided when describing GIST. Currently, doctors cannot guarantee that any particular GIST is completely benign. When calling a GIST "benign," doctors mean that the risk of spreading is very low. All but the smallest GISTs are generally thought to carry a risk of metastasis or recurrence after surgical removal.

5. What are some common myths about cancer?

The first myth is that a diagnosis of cancer is a death sentence. Some patients with GISTs are cured by surgery alone, and many others are now living long periods of time. Another belief is that the patient did something wrong that caused his or her own cancer. Although this may be true for some patients with lung cancer (caused by smoking) or liver cancer (excessive alcohol consumption), the cause of GISTs in almost all patients is unknown. There is no information currently available regarding GIST risk factors, and nothing suggests that smoking or diet increases one's risk. Another widely held myth is that if a patient with cancer undergoes an operation, the cancer will spread when the air reaches the tumor. This inaccuracy probably started when we did not have precise radiologic tests and extensive disease was often identified only at the time of an operation. Also, family members cannot "catch" a GIST. A GIST is not transmitted to family members except in exceedingly rare families in whom faulty genetic material leads to an increased risk of cancer.

Occasionally, a cell becomes capable of dividing in an uncontrolled fashion, leading to the formation of a tumor that contains abnormal cells.

Benign tumor

Although not malignant or cancerous, abnormal tissue that can grow and may even become a larger size. Unlike a cancer, a benign tumor does not invade normal surrounding tissue and does not spread to other organs.

PART TWO

More About the Biology of Cancer and GIST

What has gone wrong in a cancer cell?

What are genes, proteins, and gene mutations?

What are KIT and PDGFRA proteins? Why are they important in GIST?

More . . .

6. What has gone wrong in a cancer cell? (Broken brakes and stuck gas pedals.)

In the human body, healthy tissues and organs grow into only suitable proportions, with well-defined numbers of cells. Cancerous cells no longer recognize the body's programming to maintain balanced tissues. Some aspects of cancer's behavior resemble deranged attempts to recapture certain biological processes related to embryo development in the womb or wound healing. In contrast to normal cells, cancer cells have defective programming that leads them to act in unpredictable and destructive ways.

Our body is made up of nearly 100 trillion cells. To work harmoniously, cells communicate by sending and receiving chemical messages. Cells are "wired" internally with intricate molecular signaling pathways. This wiring network relays external messages from their surface to numerous destinations deep inside the cell in order to coordinate a proper response from the cell. In **signal transduction**, chemical messages are relayed from the cell surface into its nucleus (where **genes** are located) or into other parts of the cell. Signal transduction can switch on or switch off the activity of certain genes as needed to organize the cell's response to its environment. Cancer cells have defects in these signal transduction pathways, leading to disruption of many normal cellular activities.

Cancer researchers Douglas Hanahan and Robert Weinberg have given a list of the hallmark cancer behaviors. Tumor development is like a car that has gone out of control because of "broken brakes" and "stuck gas pedals." As adapted from *Inside Cancer: Multimedia Guide to Cancer Biology* (www. insidecancer.org/), the hallmarks are as follows:

- *Uncontrolled growth.* Cancer cells can generate their own internal signals for limitless growth. Also, cancer cells ignore signals to stop growing (*stuck gas pedals*).
- *Avoidance of death.* Cancer cells escape the signals for programmed cell suicide that normal cells obey (*broken brakes*).

In contrast to normal cells, cancer cells have defective programming that leads them to act in unpredictable and destructive ways.

Signal transduction

The internal cellular processes that relay chemical messages from the cell surface into its nucleus (where genes are located) or into other cellular compartments.

Gene

Hereditary unit on a chromosome.

- *Immortalization.* Cancer cells have a capacity to multiply over and over. Normal cells can multiply only a limited number of times (*stuck gas pedals*).
- *New blood vessels.* Cancer cells sustain the formation of new blood vessels; thus, their tumors can grow beyond a limited size (*stuck gas pedals*).
- *Tissue invasion.* Cancer cells are able to roam to distant sites in the body (*broken brakes*).
- *Evasion of the immune system.* Tumors repel or hide themselves from immune system cells that usually get rid of abnormal cells from the body (*broken brakes*).
- *Genetic instability.* Cancer cells do not carefully maintain the fidelity of their **chromosomes**. They may even acquire more chromosome abnormalities over time, whereas normal cells either repair any chromosome damage or else commit suicide as a protection for the body (*broken brakes*).

7. *What are genes, proteins, and gene mutations?*

Cancer cells have damaged genes. When someone talks about a gene, what do they mean? A gene is a part of the **DNA** that tells the cell how to make a particular **protein** (Figure 2). Each protein in the cell has a gene in the DNA that tells the cell how to make it. Every cell in an individual carries the same DNA, but only some of the genes are turned on depending on the type of cell. Damaged genes cause the cell to make defective proteins, thus leading to cancer.

Each of us has 23 pairs of chromosomes—extremely long strings of DNA that contain thousands of genes—in the nucleus of our cells. The DNA from every creature is made from the same four nucleotide bases (abbreviated A, T, C, and G). These types of bases are linked to each other to form extremely long chains. The chains of bases are what we call DNA. The **DNA base sequence** is the order of the four building blocks of the DNA (e.g., ATTCCGGA). All of the proteins of an organism are programmed with just these four bases.

Chromosome

Thread-like strand of DNA and other proteins that carry the genes and functions to provide hereditary information.

DNA

Deoxyribonucleic acid. A nucleic acid that carries the genetic information in the cell. DNA consists of two long chains of nucleotides twisted into a double helix to form chromosomes.

Protein

Large molecules made of amino acids. Proteins participate in all essential processes in a cell, and form a body's major structures.

DNA base sequence

The linear order of the four types of nucleotide bases in a DNA molecule; determines structure of proteins encoded by the DNA.

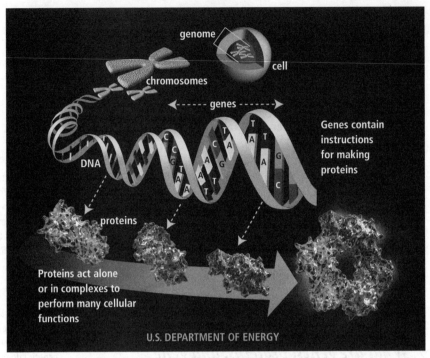

Figure 2   Cells are the fundamental working units of every living system. All the instructions needed to direct their activities are contained within the chemical DNA (deoxyribonucleic acid). Image credit: U.S. Department of Energy Human Genome Program, www.ornl.gov/hgmis.

Enzyme

Any of numerous complex proteins that are produced by living cells and assist specific biochemical reactions at body temperatures.

If genes make proteins, what do proteins do? Proteins actually perform the vital functions in the cell. Some (called **enzymes**) allow certain chemical reactions to occur or make reactions go faster; others make up the structure of the cell. In short, these enzymes allow for the chemistry that sustains life to proceed under tightly controlled conditions so that the reactions do not spin out of control. Proteins are made of smaller subunits called amino acids. When put together, proteins fold up into a specific three-dimensional shape that allows them to fulfill their mission in the cell. A protein created from a damaged gene is defective in some way. Sometimes that defective protein kills the cell, but sometimes it causes the cell to become uncontrollable and thus cancerous.

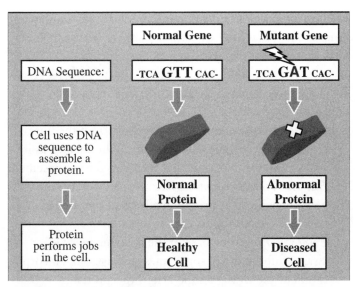

Figure 3   Any deviation from the normal DNA base sequence of a gene may lead to an abnormal protein. Abnormal proteins cause diseases such as cancer.

How does the DNA molecule serve as the blueprint from which proteins are made? This depends on the order of the four types of bases. This genetic code is "read" and then translated to make a protein. A set of three particular bases in a row is a "genetic word." This designates which of the twenty different types of amino acids is to be added next in the protein as it is being made. Amino acids are the building blocks of proteins. If one base becomes switched out for another of the bases, then the gene will be misread and a defective protein manufactured as shown in Figure 3. A gene has a **mutation** if the order of the bases within its DNA is changed from the normal sequence.

Gene mutations do not always cause serious problems; however, some mutations at critical locations within a gene can change the function of the protein so much that they lead to disease. If cell does not repair a gene mutation, then the mutation will be passed along when the cell divides to make two new cells. In this way, a single cancerous cell dividing over

Mutation

Any change in the base sequence of the DNA of a cell.

Gene mutations do not always cause serious problems; however, some mutations at critical locations within a gene can change the function of the protein so much that they lead to disease.

and over again can pass its mutations on to many subsequent generations. The results are tumors that carry the same mutations that were in the first single abnormal cell.

There are three general categories of gene mutation:

- *Deletion mutation.* Some bases are lost from the normal sequence of the gene. The protein will be smaller, as it will lack the amino acids that the deleted bases specified.
- *Insertion mutation.* Extra bases are inserted into the gene sequence. The protein made from the gene will have more amino acids than it should.
- *Point mutation.* One base in the gene sequence is swapped for another, sometimes leading to the incorporation of the wrong amino acid into a protein.

To learn more, read DNA from the Beginning (www.dnaftb. org/dnaftb/) or Human Genome Project Information (www. ornl.gov/sci/techresources/Human_Genome/project/info. shtml).

8. What are KIT and PDGFRA proteins, and why are they important in GISTs?

Defective proteins drive many types of cancers.

Defective proteins drive many types of cancers. Most GISTs contain a mutation in the *KIT* gene, whereas a few have a mutation in the *PDGFRA* gene. The *KIT* gene has the instructions for making an enzyme called KIT receptor protein, and the *PDGFRA* gene is the genetic blue print for the PDGFRA receptor protein (we use italics when describing a gene and regular type when referring to a protein [*KIT* gene versus KIT protein]). When GIST cells carry mutations in these genes, then they will make abnormal forms of KIT and PDGFRA proteins. Abnormal KIT or PDGFRA promotes several cancerous traits in GIST cells:

- Uncontrolled cell division so that tumors will grow larger

- Inhibition of pathways important for cell death so that GIST cells will not die
- Consumption of sugar at a high rate to support constant cell growth
- Migration of GIST cells to distant locations where new tumors will develop

KIT and PDGFRA are not unique to cancer cells. They are two members of a larger family of related proteins called **receptor tyrosine kinases.** Their normal forms have vital functions in many types of cells, making them beneficial for good health. When KIT and PDGFRA become defective and unregulated, they then cause harm.

Receptor tyrosine kinases
A group of cellular proteins involved in signal transduction.

The KIT and PDGFRA proteins are like "periscopes" peering out from the cell's interior space, through its membrane, and to the outside surface of the cell (see Figure 4). They are receptors for external **growth factors** arriving at the cell's outer surface. Neighboring cells secrete these growth factors. KIT becomes activated by interacting with a specific growth factor called stem cell factor. PDGFRA becomes activated by interacting with a different growth factor called Platelet-Derived Growth Factor (PDGF). As the name implies, PDGF was originally found in platelets and normally plays a role to facilitate healing wounds. The growth factors "awaken" the resting KIT and PDGFRA so that they will transmit growth signals from the outer cell surface into the interior of the cell. A cascade of events happens inside of the cell, leading to processes that support cell growth.

Growth factors
Proteins in the body that activate cells to grow.

Normal KIT and PDGFRA's pro-growth signal lasts for only a very short pulse; then it is quickly shut off. For simplicity, consider these receptors as having two alternative physical shapes or positions (Figure 4). One is the "off" position and does not send any growth signals into the cell. The other is "on." Normally these proteins idle in the "off" position until they are temporarily activated. The normal proteins never

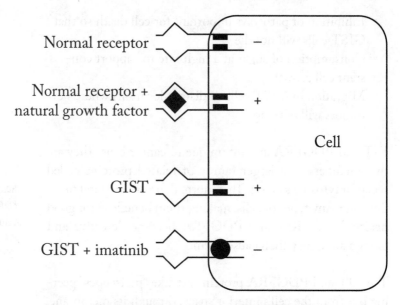

Figure 4   KIT signaling in normal states and in GIST. The KIT receptor spans the cell and relays messages from the outside of the cell to inside the cell. Normally, the KIT receptor is maintained in the "off" position. The natural ligand for KIT is called stem cell factor (shown as a diamond). When it binds to KIT, a positive signal is generated that travels within the cell. In GIST, KIT is always turned "on" even though the natural ligand is not present. Imatinib (circle) blocks KIT from transmitting a signal within a GIST cell.

spontaneously switch themselves to the "on" position in the absence of their respective growth factors.

In GIST cells, these proteins are damaged by faulty structure in a manner so they are continuously locked into the "on" position, even when their growth factors are completely absent. The result is the relentless signaling for growth into the cell. Abnormal KIT or PDGFRA send powerful messages for the cell to remain alive; thus, the only way to kill GISTs is to block these proteins. Targeted cancer therapies such as imatinib and sunitinib (see Question 57) block the signaling from these proteins and thus are effective therapies for GISTs.

9. What are primary mutations in GISTs?

When GIST is first diagnosed in a patient, research has shown that only one mutation will be detected in either *KIT* or *PDGFRA* genes from that individual, even if more than one tumor is present. Different patients are likely to have different mutations, but each individual patient's disease would only have one mutation. Most GISTs have a mutation in the *KIT* gene, whereas only a few GISTs have a mutation in the *PDGFRA* gene. These are known as the **primary mutation,** as they were present in the tumor before any treatment was initiated. The primary mutations in the *KIT* and *PDGFRA* genes tend to occur in a few specific areas of the genes ("hot spots" for mutations). To make a cell cancerous, KIT or PDGFRA proteins have to be mutated so that their altered structure is trapped in the "on" setting for cell signaling. It should not be surprising that the most common genetic mutations correlate to those parts of the protein most important for turning the protein to its "off" state. If the "off" switch is broken by mutation, then the brakes are gone, and the cancer can progress without the normal cellular growth controls.

Primary mutation

The mutations that exists in a tumor prior to any therapy.

The DNA that makes up a gene is very long, and only certain segments, called **exons**, along the greater length of the DNA are actually used to make a protein. Exons are numbered like the mile markers along a stretch of highway. They tell scientists which segment along the gene or its related part of the protein is being talked about. Scientists use the exon numbering system to report the location of a particular mutation in the *KIT* and *PDGFRA* genes. For example, the *KIT* gene is divided into 21 exons. Most of the mutations occur in exons 9, 11, 13, and 17. The sites of mutation in GISTs in the *PDGFRA* gene are in exons 12, 14, and, most commonly, 18. Figure 5 shows the overall frequencies of primary mutations for each exon for *KIT* and *PDGFRA*.

Exon

A specific portion of a gene that codes for part of a protein.

Some GISTs do not possess mutations in either the *KIT* or *PDGFRA* genes. These GISTS are "wild type" because

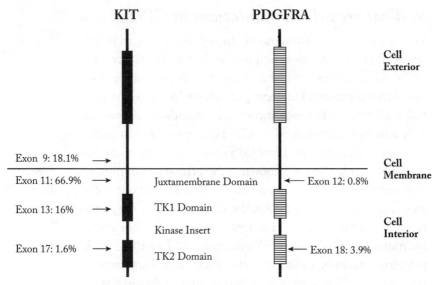

Heinrich, M. C. et al. J Clin Oncol; 21:4342-4349 2003

Figure 5   Structure of KIT and Platelet-Derived Growth Factor Receptor alpha (PDGFRA) and frequency and location of mutations in GIST. Heinrich, M. C. et al. J Clin Oncol; 21:4342–4349 2003

Neurofibromatosis

A genetic disease characterized by pigmented skin lesions, sometimes tumors that cause deformity, and predisposition to certain types of cancer.

the genes are normal. Nearly all GISTs in children, as well as the GISTs occasionally linked to **neurofibromatosis**, are the "wild-type" variety, which geneticists use to describe the normal form of genes. Mutations in some other unidentified genes likely drive these tumors.

A few GISTs test negative or are only very weakly positive for the presence of KIT protein. These are called "KIT-negative" GISTs. Most of these tumors still have a mutation in either *PDGFRA* or *KIT* gene, and thus, they can be identified even though they make little to no detectable KIT protein. An astute pathologist can see that a sarcoma-like tumor that does not stain for KIT is actually a GIST, and occasionally only sophisticated DNA testing of the tumor can truly define these as GIST.

10. Does the nature of the primary mutation affect my prognosis or treatment?

About 90% of all GISTs carry a primary mutation in either the *KIT* or *PDGFRA* genes. The presence or absence of a mutation does not necessarily determine the aggressiveness of a GIST. Early studies seemed to show a relationship between *KIT* gene mutations and aggressive tumors. We now know, however, that even small GISTs with a low risk for malignancy typically carry *KIT* mutations. In other words, a *KIT* mutation seems to be an early event in the development of a GIST. All the same, the various primary mutations are not entirely identical in their consequences. Each mutation may have a slight difference in the way that it actually stimulates the cancerous processes inside of the GIST cells. An exon 9 *KIT* mutation is found predominantly in GISTs that arise from the small intestines, whereas the various *PDGFRA* mutations occur mostly in the stomach, as do the most common GIST molecular subtype with exon 11 *KIT* mutations.

About 90% of all GISTs carry a primary mutation in either the KIT or PDGFRA genes.

A relationship exists between the location of the primary mutation and the patient's likely response to imatinib, the first therapy against inoperable GISTs. Notably, GISTs with an exon 11 *KIT* mutation have the most durable benefits from imatinib. Tumors with an exon 9 *KIT* mutation may need a higher dose of imatinib to get the same effect or might even do better with sunitinib, a recently approved drug. Because imatinib blocks the action of KIT and PDGFRA proteins, tumors without mutations in those proteins do not respond well. These "wild-type" GISTs appear to be driven by some unknown protein that the current drug therapy doesn't target. Rare primary mutations occur in the *KIT* and *PDGFRA* genes. These appear to have varying responses to imatinib ranging from fair to poor or none; although researches still lack ample data about patients with rare forms of GISTs. Table 1 summarizes some generalized characteristics of GISTs based on their primary mutation. Of course, the experience of an individual patient may differ from these overall findings.

Table 1 The characteristics of GISTs and their predicted response to the drug imatinib based on the primary mutation found in the *KIT* or *PDGFRA* genes. (Table adapted from Rubin, BP, Histopathology 2006, 48, 83–96)

Mutation Type	Frequency	Patient Response to Imatinib	Histological Type (cell shape)	Anatomical Site
KIT Gene	**80–85%**		Mostly Spindle Cell (*long and tapered*)	Entire GI tract (*except for exon 9 mutations, which are usually from the small bowel*)
Exon 9	10%	Intermediate		
Exon 11	60–70%	Excellent		
Exon 13	1%	Some*		
Exon 17	1%	Some*		
PDGFRA Gene	**5–10%**		Epithelioid (*round*) or mixed (*spindle and epithelioid*)	Usually Stomach
Exon 12	1%	Some*		
Exon 14	<1%	Unknown		
Exon 18	6%	Not Responsive		
Wild-Type (no *KIT* or *PDGFRA* mutation)	10%	Poor	Mostly Spindle Cell	

* (*few data available*)

The responsiveness of GISTs based on the type of mutation is discussed in Questions 59 and 83.

Some patients would like to know the type of primary mutation in their GIST. This is called the **mutational status** of the tumor, also known as the "tumor genotype." For a mutational analysis of your tumor's *KIT* and *PDGFRA* genes, ask your doctor. The hospital where you had surgery will have archived samples of your tumor either in paraffin-embedded blocks or as specimens on microscope slides that can be used as the material for the test. Insurance will sometimes, but not always, cover the testing. Knowing your primary mutation may eventually help your doctor recommend the optimal therapy (imatinib or sunitinib), but doctors need to learn more before they routinely use tumor genotype status to guide treatment.

11. What is tumor angiogenesis, and why is it important?

Angiogenesis (Greek word for blood vessel [angio] and birth [genesis]) occurs when the body forms new small blood vessels called **capillaries**. These capillaries distribute oxygen and nutrients to your tissues.

Adult tissues generally have all of the blood vessels they need. New blood vessels are needed only during wound healing and fetal development. Healthy tissues stop making new blood vessels at some point to stay in balance with the rest of the body. The complex steps of angiogenesis are switched on or off by a network of chemical signals that cells send to communicate with each other.

A cancer tumor also needs oxygen and nutrients from the blood. As it grows larger, an ever-expanding number of blood vessels are needed to feed the cancer cells. Many cancer cells can sustain unrestricted levels of angiogenesis. With a limitless capacity to make new blood vessels, GISTs may grow to be quite large (e.g., greater than 30 cm [about 1 foot]).

More About the Biology of Cancer and GIST

Mutational status
The type of mutation within a tumor.

Angiogenesis (Greek word for blood vessel [angio] and birth [genesis]) occurs when the body forms new small blood vessels called capillaries.

Angiogenesis
The process by which the body forms new small blood vessels called capillaries.

Capillaries
Tiny blood vessels that carry oxygen and nutrients, providing cells with the ability to grow.

The abnormal angiogenesis of a tumor involves chemical cross-talk between the cancer cells and certain normal cells that have been recruited to form the blood capillary. Many cancer cells promote this growth of tumor-feeding blood vessels by releasing a protein called **vascular endothelial growth factor (VEGF)**. This VEGF stimulates the growth of the endothelial cells required to form capillaries. VEGF released from the GIST cells combines with a receptor protein on the surface of the endothelial cells and thereby activates growth signals inside of the endothelial cell.

Anti-angiogenic therapies are supposed to interfere with this abnormal angiogenesis. A tumor cannot grow any larger without new blood vessels. Because **angiogenesis inhibitors** stop the formation of new blood vessels, they typically stabilize tumors at their current size rather than kill the cancer cells outright. **Anti-angiogenesis drugs** are used to block the signaling between the VEGF released from the GIST cells and the VEGF receptor on the capillary cells. This strategy tries to prevent GISTs from getting larger.

Vascular endothelial growth factor (VEGF)

A substance that stimulates the growth of the endothelial cells required to form capillaries.

Angiogenesis inhibitors

Substances that stop the formation of new blood vessels.

Anti-angiogenesis drugs

Same as angiogenesis inhibitors.

PART THREE

Risk Factors and Family Concerns

Who gets GIST? How common is GIST?

Did something in my environment cause my GIST?

What are the genetic risk factors for GIST?
Are my children at a higher risk for getting cancer
because of my diagnosis?

More . . .

12. Who gets GIST? How common is GIST?

GISTs are fairly uncommon. About 3,000 to 5,000 new patients develop GISTs every year in the United States. GISTs tend to occur in patients who are between 40 and 80 years old. Slightly more men than women have GISTs. The disease rarely occurs in children or young adolescents. The distribution of GISTs by race is uncertain, as large epidemiology studies have not yet been performed.

13. Did something in my environment cause my GIST?

No environmental factors appear to be associated with GIST.

No environmental factors appear to be associated with GISTs. Because of the infrequency of the disease, however, there has not been any formal study of risk factors for GISTs. In general, a large number of patients need to be analyzed to identify risk factors for any disease. Until recently, physicians could not identify large numbers of GIST patients. We will hopefully learn more about potential risk factors for GIST during the next 5 years. Currently then, an individual cannot do anything special to lessen the chance of developing a GIST.

14. What are the genetic risk factors for GIST? Are my children are at a higher risk for getting cancer because of my diagnosis?

Only a few rare genetic syndromes, such as neurofibromatosis, are associated with GIST. The chance of your children developing GIST is extremely small. Only about a dozen families in the world have been reported to have GISTs in multiple family members. Thus, nearly all patients with GIST develop the tumor spontaneously and do not inherit it from their parents. If more than one family member has GIST or a disease that may have been GIST, then genetic counseling, which your doctor can arrange, should be considered.

15. I feel like my doctors let me down because they overlooked my GIST during checkups. Are there routine screening tests for early detection of GIST?

This thought is common in a patient who is newly diagnosed with cancer. In fact, it is part of the grieving process. There are no specific symptoms that would alert your doctor to the presence of a GIST. A patient may have a very large GIST and feel fine. In most patients, blood tests are completely normal. Thus, even with your regular checkups and blood work, your doctor would not have known that you were developing a GIST. Unlike some other cancers, such as prostate cancer or liver cancer, no blood test specifically checks for GIST. Hopefully, a blood test will be developed that screens for a variety of cancers, including GIST, but this is a future research goal and remains outside of current clinical practice.

Other patients may have been experiencing symptoms; however, the diagnosis of GIST may have taken a long time because most of the symptoms are generally associated with more common conditions. For example, someone with slight stomach discomfort is much more likely to have a condition such as **gastritis** or a **hiatal hernia** with reflux than a GIST. GISTs are so uncommon that most physicians do not think of them as a cause. In fact, most physicians may never see a patient with a GIST in their entire careers.

Gastritis
Inflammation of the stomach.

Hiatal hernia
Slippage of part of the stomach from the abdomen to the chest.

PART FOUR

Diagnosis

What are the symptoms of GIST?

What are a CT scan, a PET scan, and an MRI?
Which one is best for me?

What is an endoscopy, and is it a useful
diagnostic tool for GIST?

More . . .

16. What are the symptoms of GIST?

A variety of symptoms might occur because of a GIST. Bleeding, which is common, can be very slight and even unnoticed. A doctor, using a **guaiac test**, in which a small amount of stool is placed on a special card, may detect blood in your stool. This investigation may be performed during a routine physical examination. It may be prompted by a low blood count on routine blood tests. In some cases, bleeding may be severe. Your stool may contain red blood or **melena** (dark, tarry stools). Pain is also a common symptom of advanced GIST. Actually, it is more often vague abdominal discomfort than pain, and the majority of GISTs are completely without symptoms at all.

In many patients, the GIST is diagnosed **incidentally**. Your physician may detect during examination a mass in your **abdomen**. Some patients, with even a large abdominal mass, may not notice a mass because it has developed so slowly that no abrupt change is seen. Sometimes a spouse may notice a tumor before the patient does. Some patients feel as though they have been slowly "getting fat." A GIST can also be discovered incidentally on a radiologic test such as a CT scan or an MRI or during an abdominal operation that is performed for some other reason. An **endoscopy** or **colonoscopy** may also identify an unsuspected GIST.

Fatigue, unintentional weight loss, a change in bowel habits, decreased appetite, and chronic, low-grade fevers may also be evident. These symptoms are not specific for GIST, however, and may occur with other tumors or benign conditions, such as ulcers, diverticulitis, or inflammatory bowel disease.

17. What are a CT scan, a PET scan, and an MRI? Which one is best for me?

A CT (**computed tomography**) **scan** (also called a CAT scan), which uses radiation, is a series of X-rays that provides cross-sectional images of your body. An **MRI**, using a magnetic field, also provides cross-sectional images. Although MRIs sound more appealing because no radiation is required, the small amount of radiation exposure during a CT scan is not dangerous. A patient who is claustrophobic may have difficulty with an MRI because he or she must lie still in a confined tube during the test. Patients who have metal parts in their body may not be eligible for an MRI. A patient is given a questionnaire to determine whether he or she can have an MRI.

In a CT scan and an MRI, an injection of **contrast** must be put into your vein. This, called **intravenous** contrast, makes the pictures more detailed. In addition, you will have to drink some liquid called oral contrast before a CT scan, thus allowing the intestines to be seen more easily. Typically, scans are performed of the abdomen and pelvis, as GIST commonly involves these sites.

A **PET (positron emission tomography) scan** is a nuclear imaging medicine test. A special radioactive sugar is injected into your vein; then pictures are taken to show how different parts of your body use the sugar. Many tumors, including GISTs, tend to capture the sugar faster than most normal cells. Consequently, a GIST will light up on a PET scan. A PET scan surveys the entire body. In some cases, a PET scan is done at the same time as a CT scan to provide more information. The CT performed during a PET scan may not use oral or intravenous contrast and therefore is not as good as a routine CT scan with contrast.

Your doctor will decide which test or tests to perform. In general, CT scanning provides the necessary information. If you are allergic to intravenous contrast, an MRI can be substituted for a CT. In special circumstances, or as part of a research study, a PET scan may be needed. The frequency of CT scans depends on the extent of your disease. In general, a

CT scan

Also called a CAT scan (computed tomography); a series of X-rays that are reconstructed to provide cross-sectional images of your body.

MRI

Also called MR (magnetic resonance imaging) provides cross-sectional images of the body; uses a magnetic field, instead of radiation, to generate images.

Contrast

A special type of dye that is given orally, intravenously, or rectally; the dye makes the images show up better on various radiographic studies or MRIs.

Intravenous

Through the vein.

PET scan

Positron emission tomography, a nuclear medicine test; a special type of sugar is injected into a vein, and then images are taken that show how the sugar is taken up by different parts of your body.

scan of your abdomen and pelvis should be performed every 3 to 6 months for 5 years after the removal of a primary GIST. If you have a recurrent or metastatic GIST, scans may be taken every 3 to 4 months.

18. What is an endoscopy, and is it a useful diagnostic tool for GISTs?

A gastroenterologist, a doctor who has expertise in conditions of the intestine and abdomen, generally performs the endoscopy. Endoscopy is carried out with a special scope while you are sedated. An endoscopy can be used to detect or biopsy a GIST, as long as the tumor can be reached. An **upper endoscopy** (also referred to as EGD, which stands for "esophagogastroduodenoscopy") is performed by inserting the scope into your mouth in order to examine the esophagus, stomach, and duodenum. A **lower endoscopy** (commonly known as colonoscopy) can detect abnormalities of the rectum and large colon. A GIST is different than adenocarcinoma of the gastrointestinal tract because it arises within the thick muscular wall of the gastrointestinal tract and not from the inner lining; therefore, a GIST may not be visible by routine endoscopy because the inner lining may be completely normal. If the presence of a GIST is possible, your doctor may choose to perform ultrasound (known as **endoscopic ultrasound or EUS**) during the endoscopy so that he or she can "see through" the lining of the GI tract to examine the thickness of the wall of the stomach or intestine.

19. What is a needle biopsy, and what are the risks?

As with most other cancers, the proof that you have a GIST depends on analysis of a part of the tumor. A **needle biopsy**—the insertion of a needle into a tumor to obtain a few of its cells—is examined by a **pathologist** who tries to establish the diagnosis of the **mass**. For instance, a needle biopsy helps to

Upper endoscopy
Performed by inserting a scope into your mouth in order to examine the esophagus, stomach, and duodenum.

Lower endoscopy
See colonoscopy.

Endoscopic ultrasound (EUS)
Ultrasound (using sound waves) test performed during endoscopy.

Needle biopsy
The insertion of a needle into a tumor to obtain a few of its cells for the purposes of examining the cells.

Pathologist
A physician trained in the structural and functional changes that result from disease processes; examines tissues for evidence of disease.

Mass
Often used interchangeably with tumor; sometimes the group of cells that make up a mass have an unknown origin.

determine whether a mass is a cancer. If it is, the needle biopsy reveals the type. Two types of biopsies exist: A **fine-needle aspiration** is performed by using a thin needle to obtain a few cells. A fine-needle aspiration may be performed through an **endoscope**. More commonly, a fine-needle aspiration is performed while you are having a CT scan or an ultrasound; in this case, the needle is placed directly through your skin and into the tumor. This is called a **percutaneous** (via the skin) **fine-needle aspiration**. A local **anesthetic** is injected to minimize discomfort. In contrast, a **Tru-cut biopsy** obtains a much larger sample of tissue. More tissue makes it easier for a pathologist to determine the diagnosis. A Tru-cut biopsy is performed via the percutaneous approach under CT or ultrasound guidance.

Essentially, every medical procedure or therapy has associated risks. Always ask your doctor about them. A needle or Tru-cut biopsy carries the risk of bleeding, although this is uncommon. This is particularly relevant in GISTs because they usually contain many blood vessels. Another potential risk is when a biopsy disrupts the tumor, leading to tumor spreading. Although this is a theoretical concern, it is difficult to prove that it occurs often.

In some instances, a surgeon might elect to remove a tumor without first obtaining a biopsy to establish the diagnosis. This decision is based on evidence that it is necessary to proceed directly to surgery. For instance, if the mass is highly characteristic on a CT scan, then a biopsy may not be required. In other instances, your doctor may require a biopsy before initiating treatment. Most oncologists require a biopsy before starting **chemotherapy** or drug therapy ("systemic therapy").

The tissue obtained during a biopsy is typically sent to a pathology laboratory. There it is sliced into very thin cuts that are applied to 3 × 1-inch glass pathology slides. The slices are

Fine-needle aspiration

A procedure performed by using a thin needle to obtain a few cells for examination.

Endoscope

An instrument used to examine the inside of organs, most usually the esophagus, stomach, and duodenum.

Anesthetic

A substance that is used to prevent a loss of sensation.

Tru-cut biopsy

A procedure performed through the skin to obtain a larger sample of tissue for diagnosis; performed under CT or ultrasound guidance.

Chemotherapy

Treatment with drugs intended to kill cancer cells.

stained with different chemicals that color various structures. A pathologist then examines them with a microscope, and a typed pathology report is generated. Because a very small sample of tissue is sampled, the findings may not be conclusive. In some cases, a biopsy may need to be repeated.

20. How does a pathologist diagnose a GIST?

A combination of how a GIST looks under the microscope and what proteins it expresses helps a pathologist define a tumor.

Immunohisto-chemistry

Microscopic examination of cells by staining them with antibodies.

Antibody

A protein used by pathologists to diagnose the type of a tumor.

A combination of how a GIST looks under the microscope and what proteins it expresses helps a pathologist define a tumor. In very unusual cases, examination of the tumor DNA (the tumor genotype) may be required to define the form of cancer with certainty. In many cases, a GIST has a typical microscopic appearance. Nevertheless, other tumors can have similar features; therefore, additional tests are routinely performed. **Immunohistochemistry** is used to determine what proteins are within a tumor. In immunohistochemistry, various **antibody** stains are placed on top of a specimen of your tumor. Each antibody binds specifically to a particular protein. The antibodies have colors attached to them. Tumors have characteristic patterns of proteins within them. A very useful

Pathologic Diagnosis of GIST
H&E   CD117 (KIT)

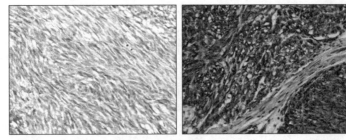

Figure 6   KIT (CD117) staining in GIST. H&E staining is shown on the left and KIT immunohistochemistry of the same tumor is shown on the right. Diffuse, strong KIT staining is typical. Magnification 40x. Courtesy of Dr. Cristina Antonescu, Department of Pathology, Memorial Sloan-Kettering Cancer Center.

marker in GIST is the protein KIT, also referred to as c-Kit or CD117. KIT is expressed in the vast majority of GISTs (Figure 6). Such tumors are KIT positive. A small percentage, called KIT-negative GISTs, does not express KIT. The diagnosis of a KIT-negative GIST is very difficult and requires an expert pathologist who may need to perform **molecular tests**, such as tumor genotyping, to make the diagnosis.

Because GIST is uncommon, some pathologists have little to no experience with diagnosing them. The results of mistaken diagnoses can be devastating, since the correct choice of treatment hinges on the correct diagnosis. It is estimated that about 5% of patients diagnosed with a GIST do not actually have a GIST. Conversely, there are also some patients who are diagnosed with other forms of cancer when in fact they actually have a GIST. Additionally, other tumors can express KIT even though they are not GIST. As stated above, the diagnosis of a KIT-negative GIST is especially difficult. If there is any question about your diagnosis, you should request that your tumor be reviewed by a pathologist at a specialty referral center with expertise in GIST.

21. Is a GIST diagnosed in children the same disease as in an adult?

No, children and young adults with GISTs have a very different type of disease. The tumors tend to occur almost exclusively in the stomach, and many are composed of cells that are **epithelioid**-shaped under the microscope (as opposed to spindle-shaped tumor cells, which are thinner and pointy in shape). Nearly all patients are female. Unlike most GISTs that occur in adults, pediatric GISTs do not have a mutation in the *KIT* gene (Question 9). Furthermore, the tumors tend to grow very slowly. Over time, the patient may commonly develop multiple tumors that arise from the stomach. Unfortunately, many pediatric GISTs do not respond well to imatinib mesylate; sunitinib's effectiveness in pediatric GISTs is under

Molecular tests

Tests of molecules essential to life such as nucleic acids and their role in genetic information.

Epithelioid

Cell morphology (shape and appearance) that looks round or polygonal.

Unlike most GISTs that occur in adults, pediatric GISTs do not have a mutation in the KIT gene (Question 9).

investigation. Because few patients have pediatric GISTs, our understanding of the disease is limited. A national cooperative effort among several major medical centers is necessary to make advances in pediatric GISTs.

There is a rare association of GIST with **paraganglioma** (a type of nerve sarcoma) and **lung chondroma** (another type of sarcoma, a benign growth of cartilage-producing cells that should not ordinarily be in the lungs). When these three tumors occur together in a single patient over time, it is a syndrome called **Carney's triad**, and it has been described as occurring in children and young adults. Most of the patients are female. The GISTs in this disease lack *KIT* or *PDGFRA* mutations and tend to arise in the stomach and may be multiple.

22. Are there different subtypes of GISTs?

As with most other cancers, **subtypes** of GISTs indeed exist. The different types of GISTs depend on their appearance under a microscope, whether they express KIT protein, or what type of genetic defect is present in the tumor cells. Microscopically, GIST cells may be **spindle** shaped (long and thin cells) or epithelioid shaped (more rounded cells), although most in adults are spindle shaped. Occasionally, a GIST contains a mixture of both cell shapes.

Nearly all GISTs express KIT protein. In fact, pathologists commonly use the presence of KIT protein to diagnose a GIST; however, up to 5% of GISTs actually lack KIT protein expression and are thus referred to as KIT negative. KIT-negative GISTs are currently not entirely understood.

The type of mutation can help to categorize a GIST. Nearly all GISTs contain a mutation in one of two genes. The *KIT* gene is mutated in most of the patients with GISTs; only a few percent have a mutation in the *PDGFRA* gene.

Paraganglioma

A type of nerve sarcoma.

Lung chondroma

A benign growth of cartilage-producing cells that should not ordinarily be in the lungs.

Carney's triad

A rare disease in young adults and children in which a GIST occurs in combination with lung and nerve sarcomas. Most patients are female. The GISTs are from the stomach, often multifocal, and lack *KIT* or *PDGFRA* mutations.

Subtypes

Different types stemming from the main type.

Spindle

Cell morphology (shape and appearance) that looks long and thin.

23. What are staging and tumor grading?

Both patients and physicians need to communicate about the cancer status; they often use certain terms that we define here. At the initial diagnosis, a primary GIST is either localized or metastatic. In a **primary localized GIST**, there is no evidence of spread to other sites. This does not mean that the tumor is benign, because even a small GIST may someday return. If a primary GIST has spread to other sites at the time of diagnosis, then it is **metastatic**. If a primary GIST has been previously removed and the tumor comes back near its original location or at a metastatic site, then it is recurrent GIST. An **advanced GIST** occurs in a patient who has metastatic disease or primary GIST that is not able to be surgically removed without causing too much harm to the normal function of the body ("unresectable" GIST). Unlike other tumors, no widely accepted staging system for GIST is available, and GISTs are not graded, although some GISTs can be called "high grade" if the cells look particularly abnormal.

24. After I am diagnosed with a GIST, what is my prognosis?

A **prognosis** is based on four general features. First, as one might expect, patients with primary disease fare better if their disease has not metastasized by the time of initial diagnosis. After a primary tumor is removed, its size, location, and evidence of its rate of cell growth allow for estimates of whether it will recur. Tumors greater than 5 cm and those that come from the intestine (instead of the stomach) have a worse prognosis, with a higher risk of recurrence. The other feature, the **mitotic rate**, is how quickly the cells within the tumor are dividing based on how they look under the microscope. The mitotic rate is typically reported as the number of cells dividing (called mitoses) in a sampling of 50 high power fields under a microscope. Your physician may estimate a risk factor for whether your disease might recur later or act malignant: low, intermediate, or high risk. Still, the prognosis for any

Primary localized GIST

The GIST tumor is found in only one place and shows no evidence of spread to other sites.

Recurrent cancer

Cancer that comes back in a patient who appeared cancer free for a time.

Metastatic GIST

A GIST that has spread to another organ or site from the primary tumor, which may or may not have been already removed.

Advanced GIST

Can refer to a patient who has metastatic disease or unresectable primary GIST.

Prognosis

Prediction of the course of an illness.

Mitotic rate

The rate at which cells divide.

given patient cannot be exactly predicted, and sometimes a patient with unfavorable tumor features can do very well, and vice versa. Table 2 shows the criteria your doctor may use to estimate your prognosis.

Table 2　Your physician will consider the size and mitotic rate of your tumor to estimate a risk factor for its potential to behave aggressively later, nevertheless the prognosis of an individual patient cannot be guaranteed by these factors. (Fletcher et al. 2002).

ESTIMATION of Malignant Potential	TUMOR SIZE Largest dimension	MITOTIC RATE Counted dividing cells in 50 High Power Fields of a microscope
Very low risk	Less than 2 cm	Less than 5 per 50 HPF
Low risk	2 to 5 cm	Less than 5 per 50 HPF
Intermediate risk	Less than 5 cm	6 to 10 per 50 HPF
	5 to 10 cm	Less than 5 per 50 HPF
High risk	More than 5 cm	More than 5 per 50 HPF
	More than 10 cm	Any mitotic rate

25. To what common locations do GISTs spread?

Peritoneum

A thin layer of tissue that covers abdominal organs.

Mesentery

Fatty tissue around the intestines.

Omentum

Fatty areas around the stomach.

The **peritoneum**, a thin layer of tissue that covers abdominal organs, and the liver are the most common sites for GISTs to spread. For instance, peritoneal tumors can develop on the surface of the stomach, intestines, spleen, or liver. GISTs can also recur in the **mesentery** or **omentum**, fatty areas within the abdomen. GISTs spread to the peritoneum through direct shedding of cells from the primary tumor. In contrast, liver metastases develop from cells that have traveled through the bloodstream. Other sites of spreading occur. Occasionally, GISTs will spread to bone or lung. Unlike many other cancers, lymph nodes are usually not involved in GIST. GISTs do not commonly spread to the lungs, or to the bones, or to the brain. Rarely, GISTs will develop again at the original location of the primary tumor. This is called a local recurrence.

PART FIVE

Coping with the Diagnosis

How can I manage my emotions? Should I take medications for either depression or an inability to sleep?

At times my outlook is not positive. Will my personality affect my chances of getting better?

What do I tell my family, friends, and/or employer? What should young children be told?

More . . .

26. How can I manage my emotions? Should I take medications for either depression or an inability to sleep?

People react differently to adverse life events. Some patients have a positive attitude, whereas others understandably cannot cope with their emotions. Patients normally require time to comprehend the scope of their problem and to identify priorities. Typically, patients first experience fear, denial, and anger. They generally fear cancer because of its uncertainty. Patients should discuss this fear with their doctors because they will feel more in control as they learn more about their disease. Patients might react with denial and anger, which should be circumvented as well. Anger might be directed against other people. This situation is very delicate, especially if those close to the patient, like family members, are also angry about the illness. Patients and their loved ones are encouraged to talk about their feelings because they need to help each other.

Depression is another common emotion for a patient who was recently diagnosed with cancer.

Depression is another common emotion for a patient who was recently diagnosed with cancer. Patients should be aware of the symptoms of depression because many of them, like loss of appetite or energy, can also occur because of the cancer. Tell your doctor that you are feeling depressed so that you can receive help. Openly discuss your feelings with your doctor. In some instances, professional help from a **psychiatrist** or other health care professional or even medications might be needed; this should be accepted as part of the healing process.

Depression

A disorder characterized by persistent sadness, sense of loss or hopelessness, sleeplessness, and/or loss of appetite or energy.

Psychiatrist

A physician specially trained in the diagnosis and treatment of mental health disorders.

27. At times my outlook is not positive. Will my personality affect my chances of getting better?

Jimmie Holland, MD, from Memorial Sloan-Kettering Cancer Center is a leading authority who knows about the special psychological needs of cancer patients. She has offered an encouraging message for those who aren't positive thinkers. When challenged with difficult circumstances, some people are naturally pessimists, whereas others are enduring optimists. For those who see the "glass as half empty," take comfort in knowing that your chances of surviving are just as good as for those who see the "glass as half full." Survival means that you seek the best medical care. Your reaction toward illness typically mirrors your attitude toward life. It is difficult to change your personality after a diagnosis of cancer comes into the picture.

Of course, people with a positive outlook might more easily feel happiness and reach out for the best quality of life after the diagnosis. Some believe in a **mind-body connection**; they use **mental imagery** to help themselves feel better about the treatments. Nevertheless, people who don't feel optimistic should not feel guilt or self-blame about their thinking. Family and friends should accept the patient's coping methods as a fundamental aspect of his or her character. Being optimistic is great, but pretending to have these feeling to please others can make you feel even more stress. Caregivers should try to notice a patient's coping style and then interact with him or her in ways that bring peace of mind and harmony.

You can find Dr. Jimmie Holland's essay "The Tyranny of Positive Thinking" at her website (www.humansideofcancer. com/).

28. What do I tell my family, friends, and/or employer? What should young children be told?

For many people, having cancer is a lonely experience. Keeping your diagnosis a secret prevents others from helping and supporting and will increase your loneliness. Although you may not currently be ready to share your thoughts and feelings, you should tell others that you appreciate their concern but are not yet ready to open a discussion. Don't push them away; reassure them that you will speak with them when you are ready. When you are ready to talk about the diagnosis,

Mind-body connection

Belief that the mind can help to heal the body.

Mental imagery

Technique used to visualize pleasant scenes in the mind; often used as a stress management tool.

When you are ready to talk about the diagnosis, decide and rehearse what you want to say. Being direct and honest is probably the easiest approach.

decide and rehearse what you want to say. Being direct and honest is probably the easiest approach.

Some friends or family members will be uncomfortable when you discuss your diagnosis. They may pull away from you—not calling or visiting as they once did. This probably occurs from their own fears about cancer or because they do not know what to say. If you don't care about this relationship, there is no reason to spend time or energy trying to reach out; however, if this relationship is valuable, call and let this person know that you miss him or her. Tell this person that you wish you could speak with or see him or her more often. Ask whether you can do anything to make him or her more comfortable. This may break the ice. Nevertheless, some people will disappoint you; however, others will surprise you because of their willingness to be helpful and supportive.

Because of fear of upsetting the children, people often try to protect children from the news that a family member has cancer; however, children can always sense when something is wrong at home, and they should hear what is happening from you rather than by overhearing or imagining something worse.

Children cope best when they are informed. Set aside time to talk with them as soon as possible after your diagnosis, and be open and honest. You may want to include the fact that you are sick and that you have cancer, the type of treatment that is planned, whether you will need to be in the hospital for a period of time, and the likely side effects of treatment and how they will affect how you look and what you will be able to do. When speaking with children, select age-appropriate language. It might be particularly helpful to practice what you want to say before starting the discussion. After the conversation, encourage the children to ask questions. Check to see that they understand what you have told them. Break down the information, and address only one or two topics at a time.

The children may ask whether you will die, or they may ask for reassurance that you will get better. Respond to their questions honestly. Tell them that you are hoping that you will be okay and that the doctor is doing everything possible. If they ask you when your treatment will be over, it is okay to tell them that you don't know. Reassure them that you will keep them informed about any changes.

Describe how your disease and treatment will affect them. Explain who will take care of them if you will be in the hospital or if you will be coming home late from a doctor's visit or treatment. Explain how your disease and treatment will affect their usual routines and activities. Be sure to ask whether they have any worries (for this answer, the authors are grateful to Eileen O'Reilly, MD, and Joanne Frankel Kelving, RN, MSN, authors of *100 Questions & Answers About Pancreatic Cancer*).

29. What are the special needs of children diagnosed with GIST?

Any child diagnosed with cancer faces many challenges. He or she is among the small percentage of those who get GIST annually. Most children with GIST are girls and are 10 years old or older, meaning that most of them have probably reached puberty, a tumultuous time for a healthy child and even more so for those with a chronic illness or a terminal cancer (Question 72 describes the treatment of GISTs in children).

First, children need to know that they did not cause the GIST. They must know that you will always be there to listen. Like any child with a chronic illness or cancer, a child or adolescent with GIST should receive honest answers to their often-difficult questions. If the child is old enough to use the computer, he or she will probably do a lot of independent research on the topic. Knowledge gives them a better sense of control, and thus, they should be welcomed into the decision-making process.

Rapidly changing emotions in your child can make coping with cancer and its treatment an especially difficult time for your family. Being sensitive to their feelings is crucial for keeping open and honest communication between family members.

We have a tendency to want to protect children; nevertheless, allowing them to attend school, interact with friends, and stay busy with normal activities is often helpful.

We have a tendency to want to protect children; nevertheless, allowing them to attend school, interact with friends, and stay busy with normal activities is often helpful. They need to talk with their friends and allow their friends to validate their feelings by saying things like "boy, cancer must really suck." When hospitalized, children can feel isolated from their friends. A special effort should be made to allow friends to visit.

Parents fear the "am I going to die?" question. Most children who have been in the medical system for a long time (GIST disease progression is slower in children), however, develop an intuition and may never ask the question. They are often more ready than their parents to consider the answer.

30. What should I know about diet and nutrition in cancer care?

Recently diagnosed cancer patients frequently ask whether any special diets will help them. Yes, good eating habits along with physical exercise can help cancer patients to feel better and stay stronger; however, there seem to be no exceptional substances in the food we eat or in the **dietary supplements** sold in stores that can change the course of the disease.

Dietary supplements

Any substance added to the diet, such as vitamins, minerals, or herbs, in addition to what the body already takes in.

Malnutrition

State of poor nutrition as a result of faulty digestion or poorly balanced diet.

The nutritional goal for patients is to maintain a desired body weight and to avoid **malnutrition**. Thus, cancer patients should select assortments of food that provide a wholesome balance of vitamins, minerals, fats, proteins, carbohydrates, and water. Nature's own intricate balance of protective nutrients as supplied by a well-balanced diet is much more preferable to supplement pills. According to the National

Cancer Institute, "Eating too little protein and calories is the most common problem facing many cancer patients. Protein and calories are important for healing, fighting infection, and providing energy."

Sometimes news reports hype preliminary and even inconclusive findings about the relationship of cancer to specific types of foods or nutrients. As a result, some may be tempted to eat particular dietary components in large amounts or to avoid them entirely. We might be lured to consume excessive dietary supplements. This strategy is wrong, as the relationship between nutrition and cancer is much more complex than that.

Cancer or cancer progression may make malnutrition worse. Advanced tumors can produce chemicals that change the way the body uses food, leading to **cachexia,** in which muscle fibers are broken down for their protein content. Advanced tumors or the side effects of treatments may cause **anorexia,** a loss of appetite. Cancer patients may face bowel blockages or debilitating diarrhea. Patients in advanced stages may have special nutritional needs that require medical intervention. Appetite-stimulating drugs are available by prescription. Patients who cannot eat by mouth may be fed using **enteral nutrition** (though a tube inserted into the stomach or intestine) or rarely **parenteral nutrition** (infused in the bloodstream).

The websites for the American Cancer Society (www.cancer.org), the National Cancer Institute (www.cancer.gov/), and the American Institute for Cancer Research (www.aicr.org) have helpful articles about the role of nutrition in cancer care, as well as tips for cooking and eating wisely. You can request an appointment with a registered dietitian from your cancer facility or primary care physician. The American Dietitian Association (www.eatright.org) assists consumers in locating a nutrition professional.

Yes, good eating habits along with physical exercise can help cancer patients to feel better and stay stronger; however, there seem to be no exceptional substances in the food we eat or in the dietary supplements sold in stores that can change the course of the disease.

Cachexia

A wasting syndrome in which muscle fibers are broken down for their protein content.

Anorexia

A loss of appetite.

Enteral nutrition

Nutrition provided though a tube inserted into the stomach or intestine.

Parenteral nutrition

Nutrition infused into the bloodstream.

31. What are some things to know about cancer-related fatigue?

Fatigue is common in people with cancer. **Cancer-related fatigue** is different from the tiredness that healthy people experience after a busy day of activities. Fatigue in cancer patients is more severe, and rest and sleep do not alleviate it. Cancer-related fatigue results from multiple chemical and behavioral factors:

- The cancer itself may release substances into the body that interfere with normal cell functions and thus cause fatigue. Some tumors secrete proteins called **cytokines** that increase your body's need for energy, weaken your muscles, and cause low-grade fevers. The metabolic waste products of tumors can act as toxins in your blood. Fatigue is commonly a symptom of **disease progression**.
- **Targeted cancer therapy** can reduce the production of red bloods cells, leading to **anemia** in some patients. Some targeted therapy drugs bring about **hypothyroidism**, a condition that slows the body's metabolic rate, leading to fatigue and sleepiness.
- Various quality-of-life factors, including pain levels, poor nutrition, nausea, sleep disturbances, and certain medications, can add to fatigue. Severe depression may also mirror symptoms of physical fatigue.

Cancer-related fatigue in some patients is mild and manageable by modifying activities, adding moderate exercise, and allowing more time for rest. For others, however, the fatigue becomes frustrating because it impairs daily performance, personal relationships, and **compliance** with treatment. Medications can treat some of the underlying causes of fatigue. For example, a skin injection of a special growth factor (**epoetin alpha**) treats anemia by stimulating the production of more red blood cells. Thyroid hormone replacement therapies alleviate the symptoms of hypothyroidism. Some oncologists

Cancer-related fatigue

Different than the tiredness experienced by healthy people after a busy day of activities; more severe and not alleviated by more rest and sleep.

Cytokines

Proteins that are secreted by tumors and increase body's need for energy; weaken muscles and cause low-grade fevers.

Disease progression

Cancer that continues to grow or spread.

Targeted cancer therapy

Treatments of drugs or other substances intended to attack cancer cells and not normal cells.

Anemia

A low level of the oxygen-containing part of the red blood cell; measured by concentrations of hemoglobin or by decreased volume or numbers of the red blood cells.

Hypothyroidism

Deficient activity of the thyroid gland.

have found that low doses of psychostimulant drugs appear to decrease fatigue, increase appetite, and promote a sense of well-being. They also counteract the sedating effects of pain-killers such as morphine; however, there are few published trials proving the effectiveness of these drugs for treating cancer-related fatigue.

32. Do complementary and alternative methods work against cancer?

Complementary and alternative medicines are outside of the realm of conventional medicine. Complementary and alternative medicines are not exactly the same. Complementary therapy is used in addition to the standard therapy. Alternative medicines are used instead of mainstream medicines and are generally not recommended in GIST.

Little is known about the usefulness of complementary and alternative methods for GIST treatment. Most complementary and alternative approaches have yet to be tested to determine safety or effectiveness. Individuals who promote the use of complementary or alternative approaches often rely on personal testimonials or anecdotal stories, which are not reliable in proving treatment effectiveness, to bolster their claims. In contrast, mainstream medicine uses scientifically designed experiments to evaluate the safety and effectiveness of new cancer therapies. The results are published in peer-reviewed journals that allow scientists and doctors to scrutinize the quality of the data and decide whether the drug seems useful. When the Food and Drug Administration approves a new drug or procedure for GIST, the therapy has met certain evidence-based criteria showing that it is beneficial.

Thus, a patient should not forgo treatment with prescription cancer drugs to use these approaches. You can safely use some complementary techniques along with standard medical treatment to improve your sense of well being:

Cancer-related fatigue in some patients is mild and manageable by modifying activities, adding moderate exercise, and allowing more time for rest.

Compliance

Act of following a treatment plan consistently and correctly.

Epoetin alpha

A drug used to treat some forms of anemia; a man-made preparation of the human growth factor erythropoietin that stimulates production of red blood cells.

Most complementary and alternative approaches have yet to be tested to determine safety or effectiveness.

- Mind-body interventions (Tai chi, Yoga, biofeedback, aromatherapy, meditation, and music therapy)
- Body manipulation methods (massage, acupuncture, chiropractic manipulation, and osteopathic manipulation)
- Biofield therapies (Reiki, Qui gong, and therapeutic touch)

Botanicals

Any plants (usually herbs or flowers) that are used as medicines.

Before using dietary supplements, such as vitamins, herbs, or **botanicals,** discuss them with your doctor. The use of supplements carries the potential for unrealized risks. Importantly, patients need to be aware of the potential for adverse drug interactions when some of these substances are combined with their cancer therapies and other prescription medications. Some botanicals can increase or slow the rates in which prescription drugs are removed from the body. If taking certain herbal supplements (e.g., St. John's wort), then you may eliminate a prescription drug from your system too rapidly to receive optimal benefit from it. Conversely, another supplement could cause you to have too much exposure to a prescription medication, thus leading to toxicities. Most producers of herbal supplements do not extensively research potential drug interactions; thus, the risks of combining them with prescription medications are unknown.

Megadosing

Excessive doses of vitamins and supplements beyond the recommended daily amount thought to improve health.

Some people believe that "natural is safe" or "natural is better," although this is not necessarily accurate. Plants are made of many chemicals—some possibly powerful or even toxic. A general multipurpose vitamin pill can be helpful if you feel as though your diet is inadequate. On the other hand, no scientific evidence shows that **megadosing** of vitamins and antioxidants is helpful—in fact, it can be toxic. Patients considering supplements should remember that "the difference between a drug and poison is sometimes the dose." Based on an understanding of how some chemotherapy drugs kill cancer cells, there is a potential of reduced effectiveness of certain chemotherapy drugs when combined with very high levels of antioxidants.

Anyone considering alternative and complementary approaches needs to be aware of the potential for **quackery**, which is the promotion of methods or products that are known to be false or unproven. Quackery generally involves soliciting a person to buy a product at expensive prices and promotes it as free from side effects or with natural healing benefits. Quackery offers junk theories about disease treatment that may even seem plausible. In fact, the claims are often erroneous if not outrageous. Some quackery practices may be harmful to the patient, and the risks may not be initially apparent to the patient. One common tactic in quackery is the promotion of products that "boost the **immune system.**" These claims again have not been scientifically tested and thus are not reliable. These are good websites to learn more about quackery: Quackwatch (www.quackwatch.org) and Canadian Quackery Watch (www.healthwatcher.net/Quackerywatch).

Quackery
Refers to the promotion of methods or products that are known to be false or unproven.

Immune system
The integrated body system that protects the body from infections and diseases.

If a complementary or alternative medicine is at some point proven to be safe and effective, then it can be adopted into conventional health care. The National Center for Complementary and Alternative Medicine (NCCAM) is the U.S. government's lead agency for scientific research on complementary and alternative approaches. It also provides fact sheets and publications to the public. The NCCAM and the National Cancer Institute sponsor various clinical trials to study complementary and alternative treatments for cancer. The NCCAM clinical trials database offers patients and health professionals information about research studies that use complementary and alternative medicine (nccam.nih.gov/clinicaltrials/). The NCCAM clinical trials database is searchable by the type of complementary and alternative therapy or the disease.

PART SIX

Financial and Work–Related Issues

What insurance and financial concerns must
I address after my diagnosis?

Why is prescription coverage so important for
GIST patients? Can I receive financial assistance
for my prescriptions?

Can I work while receiving treatment?
What should I tell my employer?

More . . .

33. What insurance and financial concerns must I address after my diagnosis?

Financial concerns are an important aspect of medical care, as health care is expensive and patients might need to stop working, at least temporarily. This might affect their insurance coverage. After being diagnosed with cancer, you should start collecting information about your health coverage options. Does the health insurance company provide only in-network coverage, thus making a patient select from the different providers and/or hospitals that his or her insurance company has an agreement with? Is an out-of-network coverage available that allows you to seek medical care where you choose? All individuals should make sure that their insurance premiums are paid and that their information is current. Document all contacts with your insurance company. Organized and well-documented information might save trouble later on. Most hospitals have a patient financial services department. To understand your rights and obligations, establish contact with this department.

Based on the severity of the illness or the extent of the treatment prescribed, you might be required to take sick leave or disability benefits, which can be done through a workplace or private insurance disability policy that may already be in place.

The government also has many helpful programs. These are divided into two big categories. Programs that are not based on income or financial means include Medicare for patients older than 65 years of age. Details can be found at www.medicare.gov. Social security (www.ssa.gov) is available for patients older than 65 years, and social security disability (www.ssa.gov) is a possibility for disabled workers and their family based on disabled status and their prior contribution to the program. U.S. veterans might also seek veterans' benefits through the Veterans Affairs Department. If you don't have the means to obtain health care, seek government support

> *Financial concerns are an important aspect of medical care, as health care is expensive and patients might need to stop working, at least temporarily.*

through Medicaid. Details about the program can be found at cms.hhs.gov/medicaid.

34. Why is prescription coverage so important for GIST patients? Can I receive financial assistance for my prescriptions?

The most effective therapies for inoperable GISTs are targeted cancer therapies. Oral cancer therapies are received through prescriptions. If you have developed inoperable GIST, you may have to remain on daily dosing of targeted cancer therapy drugs throughout the rest of your life. These drugs do not cure your tumors but rather stop them from growing. Presently, imatinib and sunitinib are the only prescription drugs that are approved for use against GIST. Both are costly name-brand drugs, and no low-cost generic alternatives are available.

Various public and private programs are available for patients who need assistance with their prescription costs. All drug-assistance programs have specific requirements that you must meet to receive assistance. The American Cancer Society (www.cancer.org) has compiled a detailed list of resources and helpful tips about drug-assistance programs.

Points adapted from the American Cancer Society are as follows:

- Pharmaceutical companies offer reimbursement programs that are usually listed at the drug's website. These programs require that you do not have an insurance plan, do not qualify for any government programs that would pay for the prescription, and have a financial hardship.
- Charitable organizations such as Patient Services Incorporated (www.uneedpsi.org) offer relief for insurance premiums and co-payments and locate options for health insurance coverage.

Presently, imatinib and sunitinib are the only prescription drugs that are approved for use against GIST.

- Information clearinghouses such as NeedyMeds (www.needymeds.com) provide information, including requirements and application forms, on hundreds of drug-assistance programs. BenefitsCheckUpRx (www.benefitscheckup.org) offers a screening service to locate programs for people who are older than 55 years.
- Government programs offer prescription coverage. Locate Medicare and Medicaid information at www.ssa.gov/mediinfo.htm.

35. Can I work while receiving treatment? What should I tell my employer?

Most patients with GIST can return to work while being treated with oral targeted cancer therapies (also known as **tyrosine kinase inhibitors**) or following surgery or other procedures to destroy tumors in specific locations (called "ablation" procedures, see Part 9). If you feel well it would probably be preferable to continue to work to keep a sense of normalcy in your life. If you are working, you are most likely entitled to sick days, or even an unpaid leave. You can check the United States Department of Labor medical leave act of 1993 at www.dol.gov/esa/regs/compliance/whd/whdfs28.htm. You may also need to review your disability benefits with the benefits department at your job.

It is natural to worry about telling your supervisor or co-workers about your cancer. The amount of information that you share is definitely a personal preference; however, you should not fear being treated differently. The American with Disabilities Act clearly states your rights and protects you against discrimination at work. It also requires that employers make reasonable adjustments as long as you can perform the essential functions of your job. You may need to discuss your work schedule, limitations, and other aspects at your department of human resources. In case of a conflict, you may need to contact your lawyer or the U.S. Department of Justice at 1-800-514-0301 or at www.usdoj.gov/crt/ada/adahom1.htm.

Tyrosine kinase inhibitors

A group of drugs that block the function of certain proteins responsible for stimulating the growth of cancer cells.

Ablation

A surgical procedure that locally destroys a tumor usually by heating or freezing.

The American with Disabilities Act clearly states your rights and protects you against discrimination at work. It also requires that employers make reasonable adjustments as long as you can perform the essential functions of your job.

Remember that your supervisor and co-workers may feel uncomfortable with your diagnosis, either because of fear or their own family experiences. Try to educate those who are interested, and remain courteous to those who shy away from you. With time, as others see that you function like any other person, their fears and anxieties may dissipate and your relationship with them may normalize.

Financial and Work-Related Issues

PART SEVEN

Getting Organized and Making Decisions

What are the best ways of managing all of the medical paperwork?

How can I most effectively communicate with my doctors?

I feel overwhelmed by all of the information that I am receiving. How do I make any decisions regarding my treatment?

More . . .

36. What are the best ways of managing all of the medical paperwork?

Be sure to keep records of all your medical reports. Get a binder to group your reports by category. For instance, you could have separate sections for diagnostic tests, blood tests, surgery, pathology reports, and doctors' notes. Having a one- or two-page summary of all the major events in your medical course, such as symptoms at presentation, date of diagnosis, method of diagnosis, surgery date and procedure, date of recurrence, dates of chemotherapy treatment and dose, and date of resistance to chemotherapy is helpful. The summary allows a physician to see your past quickly and to understand your current status better.

37. How can I most effectively communicate with my doctors?

You should communicate with your doctor openly and honestly. Because your doctor might give you a lot of information during a single visit, take a friend or family member with you, as this person may also take notes. Make sure that you understand what the doctor is saying. It can be initially difficult to focus on the facts because of the normal emotions that occur after learning of a cancer diagnosis. Become familiar with the doctor's staff, such as a nurse who can help you with basic questions. Write your questions for the next time you talk with your doctor.

38. I feel overwhelmed by all of the information that I am receiving. How do I make any decisions regarding my treatment?

This is understandable and expected. In fact, this book was written to help you manage the information about your disease. Many resources are available. Take notes but do not get caught in details, as you might lose the big picture this way. In many cancer centers, several physicians might follow your case. Your doctors will be talking to each other. Identify one physician (such as your surgeon in case you need surgery or your medical oncologist if you need chemotherapy) to be your primary caretaker.

39. How do I decide where to be treated? What is a "multimodality" approach to GIST treatment, and who will I need on my team of doctors?

Whenever possible, physicians who have experience in GIST should provide your treatment. In particular, you should be evaluated by a team of physicians (Table 3), who will usually include an oncologist and a surgeon. In addition, you may have a **gastroenterologist**, a **radiologist**, and a pathologist. Each type of doctor is vital to your care, and each has a different area of expertise. Together, they can make the best recommendations for you.

Whenever possible, physicians who have experience in GIST should provide your treatment.

Gastroenterologist

A physician specially trained in the field of diseases related to the gastrointestinal tract and organs in the abdomen.

Radiologist

A physician specially trained in the interpretation of imaging studies; a diagnostic radiologist reads conventional X-rays, CT scans, and MRIs; a nuclear medicine radiologist reads PET scans, and an interventional radiologist performs procedures.

Table 3   Multidisciplinary team of cancer specialists.

Multidisciplinary Team
DIAGNOSTIC PHYSICIANS: Pathologist Diagnostic radiologist Nuclear medicine radiologist

TREATMENT-ORIENTED PHYSICIANS:
Medical oncologist
Surgical oncologist or
   General surgeon
Specialty Surgeons such as
   • Colorectal surgeon
   • Hepatobiliary surgeon
Gastroenterologist
Interventional radiologist

Medical oncologist

A cancer specialist that specializes in the use of chemotherapy, biologic, and other nonsurgical treatments of cancer.

A **medical oncologist** is a cancer specialist that specializes in the use of drug therapy such as targeted cancer therapies, hormonal therapies, chemotherapy, biological therapies, and

Surgical oncologist

A surgeon who specializes in the surgical treatment of cancer.

Colorectal surgeon

A surgeon who specializes in colon surgery.

Hepatobiliary surgeon

A surgeon who operates on the liver and pancreas.

Pancreas

A large lobulated gland located behind the stomach and closely associated with the duodenum. It makes enzymes to digest food and regulates your blood sugar level.

other non-surgical treatments of cancer. A **surgical oncologist** is a surgeon who specializes in the surgical treatment of cancer. Other types of surgeons that you might need include a **colorectal surgeon** (specializes in colon surgery), a general surgeon (operates in multiple areas, especially within the abdomen), and a **hepatobiliary surgeon** (focuses on the liver and **pancreas**). A gastroenterologist is a doctor who deals with the health of the gastrointestinal tract, often performing procedures such as endoscopy. A pathologist has expertise in making a diagnosis from examining a tumor. There are several types of radiologists, including a diagnostic radiologist who performs and interprets CT scans and MRI scans, a nuclear medicine radiologist who performs and interprets PET scans, and an interventional radiologist who performs procedures using imaging guidance.

While working with a multidisciplinary cancer team, maintain your relationship with your primary care doctor. Although the primary care doctor may not have expertise in GIST, he or she can help to monitor you during your treatment. This is especially important if you are traveling a great distance to a cancer specialty group; it is essential to have a primary care doctor that is close by in case you need immediate care.

40. Should I get a second opinion?

Patients with cancer often obtain a second opinion, which may provide more information. Of course, different doctors may have different amounts of experience with GIST, and even experts can disagree by interpreting the same information in varying ways, and as a result, you may actually receive conflicting opinions about what you should do. Patients should try to avoid obtaining too many opinions, as this may make things more confusing or even delay critical therapy. At initial diagnosis, seeking a second opinion could be very valuable as certain therapeutic options, like surgery, might not be available at a local hospital and a patient might need to seek medical care at a larger cancer center. In patients with very advanced disease, a second opinion might help a patient decide which clinical trial to pursue. Some patients and their families might travel long distances to seek differing opinions and look for miracles. In this instance, use common sense and good judgment. More importantly, have a frank and open discussion with your physician, who is in the right position to assess the usefulness of a second opinion. Your physician may be the one who suggests a second opinion. This is not a reflection on the inability of your physician to handle the current medical situation, but rather a genuine effort to make you feel comfortable with your treatment.

In patients with very advanced disease, a second opinion might help a patient decide which clinical trial to pursue.

PART EIGHT

Management of Primary Localized GIST

How do I select a surgeon? Will I have a better outcome from a surgeon who specializes in cancer surgery?

What determines whether a tumor can or should be removed?

What are the most common surgical procedures for localized primary GIST?

More . . .

41. How do I select a surgeon? Will I have a better outcome from a surgeon who specializes in cancer surgery?

In general, you will want to be treated by someone who has experience in abdominal surgery. Because GISTs are uncommon, many surgeons may have very little to no experience and thus might not know some of the subtleties of GIST surgery. Whether you will have a better outcome by choosing a specialist has not been proven, but clearly some situations exist in which having an experienced surgeon would be beneficial.

The size and site of your tumor are also important in selecting a surgeon. A surgeon with expertise in surgical oncology and GISTs might be better able to remove a very large GIST. For instance, a small tumor in the small intestine or at the end of the stomach is often easily removed and can be performed by most general surgeons. A colorectal surgeon or someone with considerable expertise in rectal surgery should perform removal of a low rectal tumor.

42. What determines whether a tumor can or should be removed?

Several factors determine whether a GIST can be removed:

1. *Whether the tumor is primary or metastatic.* First, it is important to determine whether you have a primary localized GIST or a primary GIST with metastasis. In general, the **preoperative** CT scan can determine this; however, metastasis is occasionally discovered during an operation, leading to the termination of the procedure without tumor removal. If the tumor has already spread, your doctor may want to treat you medically first, even if all of your disease is technically removable.
2. *Your general health.* You should be in adequate general health to tolerate anesthesia and the required surgi-

---

Whether you will have a better outcome by choosing a specialist has not been proven, but clearly some situations exist in which having an experienced surgeon would be beneficial.

Preoperative

Before surgery.

The type of surgery that you need depends on the location of your tumor and involvement of surrounding structures.

---

cal procedure. For instance, if you have a weak heart, attempting a resection of your GIST may not be advisable. In that case, your doctor may treat you with medical therapy.

3. *The relationship of your tumor to vital structures.* Certain structures in the body, such as certain blood vessels, cannot be removed. In general, GISTs tend to push surrounding structures without invading them. Nevertheless, a GIST may become inseparable from an adjacent vital structure. This may be determined based on radiologic tests or at the time of surgical exploration. In this case, your doctor may want to treat you medically first and then attempt removal of the tumor later.

43. What are the most common surgical procedures for localized primary GISTs?

The type of surgery that you need depends on the location of your tumor and involvement of surrounding structures. The most common procedures are partial **gastrectomy** (partial stomach removal) or partial intestine **resection**. A total gastrectomy is rarely necessary. Other organs that must sometimes be removed include the left portion of the pancreas and the **spleen**. An **abdominoperineal resection** may be required for a tumor that is close to the end of the rectum. In this case, a permanent colostomy is needed. Some tumors in the duodenum might require a **pancreaticoduodenectomy**, also called a **Whipple procedure**. In this operation, part of the pancreas, a small piece of intestine, possibly part of the stomach, part of the bile duct, and the gallbladder are removed. Your doctor will explain what must be sacrificed to remove your tumor.

44. How do I prepare for surgery?

After you and your doctor decide that removal of your tumor should be attempted, certain preparations will be made. If you are older or have certain medical problems, you might need to see a general medicine doctor or a **cardiologist** to determine whether you are healthy enough for an operation. You might

Gastrectomy
Removal of the stomach.

Resection
Surgical removal of an organ or other body structure.

Spleen
A highly vascular abdominal organ that filters the blood and contributes to the immune system.

Abdominoperineal resection
Removal of the rectum and anus.

Whipple procedure
Operation in which part of the pancreas, a small piece of intestine, possibly part of the stomach, part of the bile duct, and gallbladder are removed. Also called pancreaticoduodenectomy.

Cardiologist
A physician specially trained to care for patients with heart problems.

Stress test

A test that measures heart function during strenuous exercise or after medication is given.

Echocardiogram

An ultrasound of the heart that examines its structure and function.

Electrocardiogram

ECG or EKG, tracing of the electrical impulses of the heart.

Anesthesiologist

A physician who is specially trained to administer anesthesia during surgery.

even be asked to undergo certain tests, for example, a **stress test** or **echocardiogram**.

Next, preadmission testing will be done, including routine blood tests, an **electrocardiogram**, and a chest X-ray. This is standard before undergoing general anesthesia. Often, you will also meet an **anesthesiologist**. In most cases, patients will be admitted the day of the operation. If special medical circumstances are present, you might be admitted to the hospital one or a few days before the operation. Depending on the location of the tumor, the surgeon may have you take some medication to clean out your intestines.

On the morning of surgery, do not eat or drink. Your physician will have told you whether to take your normal medications with a sip of water. You will be asked to arrive at the hospital several hours prior to the time of the operation, possibly as early as 6 a.m. You will be asked to get undressed and to put on a hospital gown. Patients will generally be kept in a holding area, sometimes with family members, until the operating room is ready. Several different people will likely ask you your name, the name of your doctor, your medical history, the intended surgical procedure, and your allergies. Although such repetition might become annoying, it helps to ensure your safety.

Ultimately, you will be taken into the operating room. You will meet several nurses, surgical assistants, an anesthesiologist, and the surgeon. The operating room is often somewhat cold, but you will have several blankets during the operation. An intravenous (IV) will be started in your arm if not placed already in the holding area. You will be placed flat on a table, and anesthesia will be administered.

45. What happens during surgery for GIST?

After you are asleep, someone will shave the hair on your belly (if necessary). Your belly will then be washed with soap.

Generally, a small tube, called a **Foley catheter,** will be placed into your bladder so that the amount of urine can be closely monitored. A larger IV may be placed into your neck to give more fluids and/or medications that might be needed for support through the operation.

In some circumstances, with the patient under anesthesia, the surgeon may decide to perform a **laparoscopy** immediately before opening your abdomen. With this, a few small incisions are made in order to insert a telescope and some instruments. Specifically, the surgeon is looking to see whether the cancer is more advanced than what is shown on the radiologic tests. In some cases, the entire operation can be performed using only laparoscopy.

A number of different **incisions** can be used to open an abdomen (see Figure 7). The most common is a midline incision. Alternatively, an incision can be made under on or both rib cages. Your surgeon will decide whether your tumor can be removed. Although a tumor may seem removable on a CT scan or MRI, this may not actually be accurate. The surgeon might find that the tumor cannot be removed because it has spread or because it is connected to vital structures.

Foley catheter

A narrow tube placed in the bladder so that the amount of urine can be closely monitored.

Laparoscopy

Performed under general anesthesia; a few small incisions (less than an inch) are made in order to insert a telescope and some instruments in order to inspect the organs of the abdomen and/or pelvis.

Incisions

Surgical cuts in the skin.

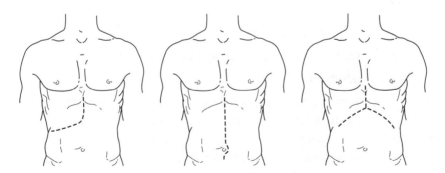

Figure 7   The most common surgical incisions are shown by the dotted lines. The middle drawing shows the most common approach although the length may vary. The other 2 incisions are used for liver resections or upper abdominal surgery. Reprinted with permission of Memorial Sloan-Kettering Cancer Center.

Blood transfusion

The procedure to replace or augment a person's volume of blood.

Pneumonia

A disease of the lungs that is usually caused by infection. It is accompanied by fever, chills, cough, and difficulty in breathing.

Pulmonary embolus

A blood clot that lodges in the lung.

A loss of appetite is common immediately after surgery; if you recover from the operation without major complications, your appetite should return within a few weeks.

Vitamin B₁₂

A vitamin needed to treat pernicious anemia, a form of anemia resulting from stomach disturbances that prevent the absorption of B₁₂.

46. What are the risks of surgery?

The risks of surgery are related to anesthesia and the actual removal of the tumor. Anesthesia carries the risk of heart attack and stroke. The chance of dying from anesthesia is usually less than 1%.

The general risks of abdominal surgery include bleeding, especially for larger GISTs. A **blood transfusion** may be necessary. A patient rarely needs to go back to the operating room for bleeding that occurs after the operation. Typically, the part of the gastrointestinal tract where the GIST arises needs to be removed; thus, there is a small chance that there will be leakage of gastrointestinal fluid from where the tumor is removed. Other complications include infection in your urine from the catheter. **Pneumonia** is another risk. Occasionally, the abdominal incision does not heal completely, and the wound may need to be packed with gauze for about a week after the operation. Uncommonly, a patient will develop a blood clot in his or her leg from being relatively inactive. This is sometimes treated with a blood-thinning medication. The worst scenario is a blood clot that breaks free and goes to the lungs. This—called a **pulmonary embolus**—can be life threatening.

47. How will removal of parts of my stomach or sections of my intestines affect my digestion?

Your doctor will explain how the surgery may alter your digestive function. A loss of appetite is common immediately after surgery; if you recover from the operation without major complications, your appetite should return within a few weeks. If a large part (or all) of your stomach is removed, then you may need a special diet that includes small, frequent meals. You can live a normal lifespan without a stomach. You will need to take certain supplements including **vitamin B₁₂** shots. **Dumping syndrome,** in which you have diarrhea and skin flushing after eating a meal, is a potential complication of removing the stomach. This is generally treated with diet modification. You might need to speak with a nutritionist.

Diarrhea may occur if you lose a large part of either the small or large intestine. Occasionally, a patient requires a temporary or permanent colostomy after tumor removal.

Adhesions are scar tissue that develop after most abdominal operations. Similar to a deep cut on your arm, if you undergo abdominal surgery, some scar tissue will form. Some patients have only a little scar tissue, whereas others have a lot. There is no way to predict this. A few people will form enough scar tissue to block their intestines at some point in the future. This—called a **bowel obstruction**—may resolve with bowel rest and not eating, or it may require an operation. Most patients with bowel obstruction will develop crampy, abdominal pain and possibly vomiting.

48. How fast will I recover immediately after surgery and in the days that follow?

After the operation, you will be taken to a recovery room for observation. Bleeding is the main immediate risk after surgery. A patient may rarely need to undergo an emergency operation to control bleeding. Depending on the hospital and the extent of your operation, you may stay in a highly monitored setting for a few days, or you may be transferred directly to a regular patient floor. Overall, expect to be in the hospital for up to 7 to 10 days. If everything goes well, you should be able to sit in a chair, and in most cases walk, the day after your surgery. You should be ready to eat again after a few days. When you start eating, you may get full quickly. Unless you had a large part or all of your stomach removed, this should get better over several weeks. Also, initially, a decreased appetite is normal after an operation. A special intravenous pump that you control provides the pain medication. The nurse will teach you how to use it. Pain is generally the worst in the first few days

Dumping syndrome

A potential complication of removing the stomach in which diarrhea and skin flushing are present after eating a meal; generally treated with diet modification.

Colostomy

The surgical construction of an artificial opening into the colon that allows fecal material to empty into a bag.

Adhesions

Scar tissue that develops after most abdominal operations.

Bowel obstruction

Condition in which the intestines do not function properly because something is blocking them from emptying.

after surgery. By the time you go home, you may need only a small dose of pain medication or even none at all.

After discharge from the hospital, expect to recover completely over the next 3 to 6 weeks. You will slowly regain your energy. Although you may not see improvement each day, you should notice that each week you are feeling better. If not, notify your doctor. Also, notify your doctor if the incision turns red, if leakage develops through the wound, or if you have fever. Usually, if your doctor agrees, you can drive in a few weeks, when pain medication is no longer necessary. You should not do any heavy lifting for several months so that you do not disrupt the incision. A wound actually takes 6 to 12 months to heal completely. Most importantly, you should regain your quality of life in almost all cases.

49. Am I cured if the surgical team says "we got it all"?

Cured means that your tumor never comes back. Although it is satisfying to hear from your surgeon that all of the tumor was removed, you are not necessarily actually cured. This does mean, however, that the surgeon removed all of the visible disease. Some patients develop tumor recurrence because residual microscopic disease exists that cannot be detected and therefore cannot be treated. No test can currently detect microscopic disease. For instance, a few cells might spread from the primary tumor to somewhere else in the abdomen, like the peritoneum or the liver. These would not be seen at surgery. Radiologic tests can detect tumors that are only about a quarter of an inch or larger. In general, no one can definitively predict whether your GIST will return; however, if it is a very small tumor, you probably are truly cured.

Doctors normally measure the outcome of patients with cancer by determining what percentage will be alive at 5 years. Again, doctors generally cannot reliably predict what will happen to any given patient. This can be compared with grades in school: The average grade in a class may be a "C," but some patients do a lot better and others a lot worse. The application of tyrosine kinase inhibitors to GISTs has dramatically improved outcome, as discussed in Questions 57 and 58.

50. What is done with my tumor after it is removed? What is in the pathology report? Does the hospital save any part of my tumor, and will I need these samples?

The tumor and normal tissue that your surgeon removes are sent to a pathologist, who will examine the specimen with a microscope. Special tests (called immunohistochemistry) that see whether certain antibodies bind to your tumor will be performed (as discussed in Question 20). One such antibody detects CD117 or KIT. If the antibody binds, your tumor expresses a certain protein, in this case KIT. Almost all GISTs are KIT positive.

The pathology report contains a lot of information and will state the size and number of tumors. The pathologist also determines whether the surgeon achieved a **negative margin of resection** by entirely removing the tumor with a rim of normal tissue around it. If lymph nodes were removed, the report will state whether tumor cells existed in them. In GIST (except for pediatric GIST), lymph nodes generally do not need to be removed because the GIST rarely travels there. If any nodes are enlarged, the surgeon may remove those. The pathologist also determines the site where the tumor arose, as this sometimes may not be clear to the surgeon. The pathologist also determines how actively the tumor was dividing when it was removed.

The pathologist stores part of your tumor in paraffin wax and may also freeze some of it. The rest is discarded. You should be able to access the stored samples in the future, as they are sometimes needed if you change doctors or go on to participate in a clinical trial, in which case another doctor

The pathology report contains a lot of information and will state the size and number of tumors.

Negative margin of resection

No cancer cells are found in the edge of the surrounding tissue that's removed along with the tumor.

may want to confirm that your tumor was in fact a GIST. An expert sarcoma pathologist might be needed to examine the tissue directly if the diagnosis is in doubt. Your doctor might also want your tumor to be analyzed for its mutation status (Question 10).

Surgical margins

The amount of normal tissue that the surgeon removed around the tumor.

In general, a surgeon always tries to get negative margins; however, this is not always possible if the tumor was in a particularly difficult area, if a larger resection could not be performed without causing potential harm to the patient, if a larger resection could not be performed because of the involvement of vital structures, or if the patient does not agree to a large resection.

51. What are surgical margins, and how do they affect my outcome?

Surgical margins are the amount of normal tissue that the surgeon removed around the tumor. The pathologist will estimate this amount of tissue. In particular, the pathologist will look microscopically to determine whether there is tumor at the microscopic margin. In general, a surgeon always tries to get negative margins; however, this is not always possible if the tumor was in a particularly difficult area, if a larger resection could not be performed without causing potential harm to the patient, if a larger resection could not be performed because of the involvement of vital structures, or if the patient does not agree to a large resection. The actual width of the negative margin does not appear to be important as long as it is negative. If you have a positive microscopic margin, then your chance of having the tumor come back may be higher. If your surgeon could not remove all of the visible tumor, then other treatments will need to be considered.

52. Should I receive adjuvant therapy to prevent recurrence of my primary localized GIST? What is neoadjuvant therapy?

Adjuvant therapy is the use of chemotherapy, radiation, or any other form of treatment given after surgical removal of cancer. In some types of cancer, chemotherapy is routinely given after tumor removal. This hopefully kills any microscopic cancer cells that remain, thus preventing the recurrence of the cancer. Currently, however, the standard of care after GIST removal is simply patient observation, which means undergoing routine radiologic imaging and physical examination by your doctor. Clinical trials are testing whether adjuvant use of tyrosine kinase inhibitors improves survival after the resection of primary GIST.

In some cases, a surgeon cannot remove a GIST because of its large size or close proximity to vital structures so that surgery would inflict too much damage to the normal functioning of organs. In other cases, removal of the tumor may require a large sacrifice of normal tissue and risk severe impairment to the quality of life of the individual. For such patients, the GIST is considered functionally "unresectable," since surgery would be unacceptably risky, and the recommendation might be for you to receive targeted cancer therapy rather than surgery. Some might consider this "neoadjuvant" therapy, which is chemotherapy administered prior to surgery, because it might be possible to shrink the tumor and allow the surgeon a chance to remove it safely, reducing the risk of the operation, or decreasing the amount of normal tissue that needs to be sacrificed. For instance, neoadjuvant therapy may be used to convert an operation from total removal of the stomach to a partial removal of the stomach, which would give the patient more normal eating capability. Or, to avoid the need for a permanent colostomy, therapy to shrink a tumor that would be considered unresectable without disfiguring surgery may be given for a low rectal tumor.

Adjuvant therapy is the use of chemotherapy, radiation, or any other form of treatment given after surgical removal of cancer.

At the current time, such pre-operative therapy with the intent to shrink tumors that are considered "unresectable" is generally performed by giving the patient imatinib mesylate (discussed later) for 1 to several months. Other agents are likely to be tested soon. Your doctor will determine whether the neoadjuvant therapy is working (shrinking the tumor) by performing follow-up radiologic tests. It may even take up to a year for a tumor to shrink, and so it is appropriate for both you and your doctor to be patient as long as the GIST is not obviously growing or getting worse in some way.

53. What types of routine imaging procedures, laboratory tests, and checkups are necessary after my surgery? For how many years will I need to be monitored?

Patients should be monitored with radiographic tests at routine intervals after removal of a primary GIST. A helical CT scan of the abdomen and pelvis with oral and intravenous contrast is preferred. An alternate test is an MRI of the abdomen and pelvis with intravenous contrast (oral contrast is not used with an MRI). Your doctor might perform standard laboratory tests once or twice per year. Patients should be followed with a scan every 3 to 6 months for at least 5 years because a patient has the greatest risk of recurrence within 5 years of the original operation. Occasionally, a patient's tumor may come back after 5 years, so periodic scanning may also be medically indicated even after 5 years, depending on the risk assessment of the original tumor.

PART NINE

Medical Therapy of Metastatic GIST

What does it mean to have a metastatic GIST?

If I have a metastatic GIST, can I be cured with drug therapy? How long will I need to be on targeted cancer therapy?

Targeted cancer therapies are promising new methods for treating cancer. How do these drugs differ from traditional forms of chemotherapy?

More . . .

54. What does it mean to have a metastatic GIST?

GISTs are either diagnosed as primary localized tumors or metastatic GIST. Metastatic GIST means that a primary GIST tumor has spread to other parts of the body. The outcome for GIST patients who have recurrence of their disease (which means that the tumor has come back at its original location after surgical resection of the primary tumor) appears to be similar to patients with metastatic GIST that has spread, and so often metastatic and recurrent disease are considered similarly for consideration of therapy. Metastatic GIST most commonly involves the liver or the peritoneum, the thin layer of tissue that forms the lining and covering for the abdominal organs. Because the peritoneum covers multiple organs (including the stomach, intestines, and abdominal fat), GIST can spread to any of these areas. GIST can also move into the pelvis, which is a very small area that can be difficult for surgeons to completely remove tumors. GIST is rarely able to spread to the lungs or bones. If a patient has spread of a cancer to lung and nowhere else, it may not be a GIST at all, and it may be some other form of cancer that has been mistaken for a GIST. Many other cancers spread to lymph nodes but this is usually not the case with GIST. GIST spreads to the liver using the bloodstream. Only about 25% of patients have metastases at the initial diagnosis of a primary GIST. It is exceedingly rare for GIST to spread to the brain or the spinal cord.

Metastatic GIST means that a primary GIST tumor has spread to other parts of the body.

55. If I have a metastatic GIST, can I be cured with drug therapy? How long will I need to be on targeted cancer therapy?

Being "cured" means that a tumor never returns. Although current targeted cancer therapies can control the disease for years at a time and even drastically reduce the size of the tumors, metastatic GIST is rarely (if ever) completely eradicated. The targeted cancer therapy results in complete disappearance of a tumor in only less than 5% of patients and even these patients may not be truly cured as microscopic cells may still exist somewhere. The combination of medical therapy followed by surgery may also leave you with no visible tumor, but again it is not clear that you are cured. In fact, medical therapy is usually resumed after surgery for metastatic GIST to reduce the likelihood of subsequent tumor recurrence, since a randomized clinical trial has shown that GIST patients who stop targeted cancer therapy following even complete disappearance of their disease have an unacceptably high risk of having the disease come back within weeks to months after stopping the treatment.

Nearly all patients with metastatic GISTs should be treated first with tyrosine kinase inhibitor therapy. Currently, imatinib is tried first, and sunitinib is used if imatinib fails or cannot be tolerated. Rarely, a patient with a metastatic GIST may be treated with surgery first if he or she has severe symptoms from recurrent tumors or limited metastatic disease. Your doctor will discuss your options with you based on the specifics of your case.

In order to retain control of the disease, targeted cancer therapy (either imatinib or sunitinib) may be continued for as long as you live or for as long as you can tolerate the therapy. If symptoms cannot be controlled by lowering the dose, the drug may be temporarily stopped, the symptoms treated with other medication, and targeted therapy discontinued. Withdrawing targeted therapy can cause a sudden increase in the size of existing tumors. Your physician will need to weigh the benefits of the targeted therapy versus any side effects that you may experience from the drug therapy.

In many patients, most GIST cells die or at least become inactive when tyrosine kinase inhibitor drugs such as imatinib or sunitinib block their abnormal KIT protein; however, even when the tumors look completely dead on radiologic tests, small numbers of GIST cells almost always remain.

Fortunately, these "sleeping" GIST cells can remain dormant for long periods of time. These residual cells can eventually start growing again, however, and that is why you need to be carefully monitored while on therapy.

56. Targeted cancer therapies are promising new methods for treating cancer. How do these drugs differ from traditional forms of chemotherapy?

Traditional chemotherapy drugs kill cancer cells typically by interfering with structures that are shared by normal cells as well as cancer cells. These include structures like DNA (the genetic code material that is found in chromosomes) or microtubules, the internal "tie lines" that keep cells together. Because cancer cells usually are not as "smart" as normal cells and cannot repair themselves when they are damaged as well as normal cells, they tend to be somewhat more sensitive to chemotherapy than normal cells. However, some normal cells are also very sensitive to chemotherapy. Because traditional chemotherapies are not very specific to the precise defects making cancerous cells different from normal cells, these drugs may cause considerable side effects to patients.

Apoptosis

One way in which cells die after being exposed to chemotherapy.

Actually, traditional chemotherapy doesn't kill cancer cells directly, but rather it inflicts enough damage on the cells to stimulate their internal self destruction mechanisms. This cell suicide process is known as **apoptosis**. It cuts up cells by a controlled series of events, and it is how cells die after being exposed to chemotherapy. Some types of cancer cells have become so deranged that they are no longer able to destroy themselves by their own internal programming for apoptosis. As a result they are not susceptible to the chemotherapy. GISTs are notoriously resistant to all forms of traditional chemotherapy drugs. The abnormal KIT protein within GIST cells sends continuous signals for them to survive no matter what. Only by shutting off the abnormal KIT protein are the GIST cells able to undergo cell death.

Basic scientific research over the past two decades has brought significant advancements in our understanding of how cancer develops based on molecular abnormalities within a cell. Scientists are now designing drugs that rationally take aim at those specific abnormal genes and their associated proteins that drive the growth of cancer. These new targeted cancer therapies selectively act on the traits of cancer cells that make them different from normal cells, thus sparing normal tissues. This new class of drugs is sometimes called **molecular-targeted drugs** or **molecularly targeted therapies,** because these drugs work precisely against particular abnormal molecules within a type of cancer. Some targeted therapies are given to patients by vein, but many are administered as an oral pill.

Molecular-targeted drugs or molecularly targeted therapies

Drugs that work precisely against particular abnormal molecules within a type of cancer.

Targeted cancer therapy has revolutionized the treatment of GIST. Just 10 years ago, most patients with metastatic GIST would die of their disease between 12 and 18 months on average. Nowadays, the average lifespan is nearly 5 years from the diagnosis of metastasis. In fact, imatinib and sunitinib have made GIST, even though it is an uncommon cancer, a model for all other solid tumors, representing the major clinical benefits that can be derived from a deep understanding of what makes specific cancer cells "tick."

There are several categories of targeted cancer therapy drugs that oncologists use today, although not all of these are used for GIST patients at the present time. Examples include:

Signal transduction inhibitors

Small molecules which interfere with cell surface receptors that relay growth signals from the environment into the cell; may also inhibit proteins within cells that speed up the chemical reactions for growth.

- *Signal Transduction Inhibitors.* These small molecules interfere with cell surface receptors that normally function to relay growth signals from the environment into the cell. When these are mutated, though, they can get "stuck in the ON position" and cause the equivalent of a "short circuit" inside the cancer cell. Signal transduction inhibitors may also inhibit certain proteins (called enzymes or kinases) within cells that speed up the chemical reactions for growth. The most common cellular targets for signal transduction inhibitors are enzymes

Receptor tyrosine kinases

A group of proteins on the cell surface involved in signal transduction.

classified as **receptor tyrosine kinases.** Abnormalities in certain protein kinases are relatively important to several different forms of cancer. Drugs that block the activities of receptor tyrosine kinases are classified as "kinase inhibitors."

- *Monoclonal Antibodies and Biological Therapy.* Biological therapies use antibodies, cytokines, and other immune system substances produced in the laboratory to alter the interaction between the body's immune defenses and the cancer cells. Cancer vaccines encourage the body's immune system to recognize a few types of cancers and this has been mainly studied in **melanoma** so far.

Melanoma

A form of skin cancer that can begin as a mole or a darkly pigmented area on the skin.

- *Cell-death-inducing drugs.* Many cancers protect themselves by counteracting pro-death signals. These types of drugs promote cell death by interfering with proteins that normally act as regulatory counterparts against pro-death signals.

- *Angiogenesis inhibitors.* Tumor growth relies on the formation of new blood vessels from healthy, surrounding tissue (angiogenesis). By inhibiting the growth of blood vessels in a tumor, angiogenesis inhibitors starve tumors of a blood supply, blocking their ability to grow (see Question 11). These drugs may also affect the leakiness of blood vessels and may increase the delivery of drug therapy to tumors to improve their effectiveness.

- *Gene therapy.* Cancer cells may be missing certain genes or have too much of other genes. Gene therapy attempts to correct those errors. Viruses can deliver a gene into a cancer cell, and this new information then becomes part of the cell's genetic make-up. **Antisense therapy** works much like a zipper at the genetic level to stop the process by which cancer-causing proteins are produced.

Antisense therapy

Synthetic genetic material that may stop or slow the growth of cancer cells.

57. What kinase inhibitors are important for treating metastatic GISTs? What is imatinib?

Imatinib mesylate (Gleevec™) is the first targeted therapy that is used in patients with unresectable primary GIST or metastatic GIST. The drug is approved by the U.S. Food and Drug Administration (FDA) for KIT-positive GIST, which means that a pathologist can find KIT protein on the surface of the GIST cells. However, it should be emphasized that there are at least two problems with this: first, it can be difficult in some GISTs to find KIT, since it may only be present on a few percent of the cells in a large tumor. Second, studies have shown that imatinib may be effective in a subset of KIT-negative GISTs since they too might contain a KIT or PDGFRA mutation. Imatinib is also effective in **chronic myeloid leukemia (CML)** and the FDA first approved this drug for use in this cancer of the blood (because imatinib blocks another mutant kinase enzyme inside the leukemia cells called BCR-ABL).

Imatinib is a tyrosine inhibitor that blocks the function of abnormal KIT and PDGFRA proteins which may occur in GIST. As discussed in Question 8, KIT protein in GIST is locked in the "on" position and thus sends too many signals for the cell to survive, grow, and spread. Imatinib halts these abnormal signals resulting in tumor stabilization or shrinkage in up to 85% of patients. When tumor shrinkage occurs, most of it takes place within the first 6 months of therapy (although it may continue beyond that as well). Although imatinib has been labeled as a "magic bullet," it is important to recognize that it rarely results in complete tumor disappearance.

Due to the success of imatinib therapy in metastatic GIST, several clinical trials are currently ongoing to see whether or not it might also be useful to improve outcomes of patients after complete resection of a primary localized GIST. The idea is to reduce the chance of the tumor coming back in these patients. The trials compare patients who receive adjuvant imatinib to those who receive **placebo** after surgery (since

Imatinib mesylate is the first targeted therapy that is used in patients with unresectable primary GIST or metastatic GIST.

Chronic myeloid leukemia

A slowly progressing disease in which too many white blood cells are made in the bone marrow.

Placebo

An inactive substance that contains no medication or active ingredient to be given to participants in a clinical trial to determine the effectiveness of a particular medication or substance given to other participants.

only close follow-up without any drug therapy is the current standard of care for patients with primary localized GIST following complete resection). The results of these trials should become available in the next few years.

Because imatinib is a somewhat costly medication, the manufacturer of imatinib (Novartis) can provide you with a financial hotline where reimbursement specialists can help you with your questions about insurance, billing, and financial assistance. You can learn more from the manufacturer's official website for Gleevec™ (see Question 34).

58. Are anti-angiogenesis drugs good treatment options for GIST? What is sunitinib?

Sunitinib (Sutent™) is another kinase inhibitor that has been approved by the FDA for care of patients with metastatic GIST following failure of imatinib. Similar to imatinib, sunitinib blocks the actions of both KIT and PDGFRA. However, sunitinib blocks many other signaling kinases too. Sunitinib functions as a very potent anti-angiogenic agent or angiogenesis inhibitor. By inhibiting all three forms of the Vascular Endothelial Growth Factor Receptors (VEGFR1, VEGFR2, and VEGFR3), sunitinib inhibits the formation of new blood vessels around the tumor, which the tumor needs before it can grow larger. Sunitinib is also highly effective in treating kidney cancer because that very vascular form of cancer relies on overactive signals through the VEGF receptors.

Sunitinib is currently approved by the FDA for use in GIST patients who either have developed tumors resistant to imatinib, or who cannot tolerate the side effects of imatinib. At present (2006), sunitinib is a "second line of defense" therapy for GIST after imatinib is no longer helpful to the patient. A recent clinical trial was stopped prematurely when the tumors in patients taking sunitinib had significantly longer periods of disease control (no further growth of their tumors) than did patients taking nothing (placebo). The patients taking sunitinib also tolerated it reasonably well overall with manageable side effects. In the trial, the patients on placebo who had significant growth of their tumors were immediately offered the chance to start sunitinib.

The manufacturer of sunitinib (Pfizer) also offers a financial hotline where reimbursement specialists can help you with your questions about insurance, billing, and financial assistance.

59. How does my doctor decide the drug or dose best for me?

Clinical studies establish the drug dose that seems to work well for most patients. This is the called the standard dose. Some patients may need to take more than the standard dose to control their tumors, although the higher doses often have more unpleasant or even medically threatening side effects. Other patients may require a lower dose because of the side effects; however, lowering your dose past a certain threshold may result in less ability of the drug to control your cancer. The optimal dose of a cancer drug is generally a compromise between the benefits of higher amounts of the drug to stop your tumors versus the increased risks for adverse side effects at these higher doses.

The starting dose of imatinib is usually 400 mg daily, but some physicians may choose to use 600 or even 800 mg daily, based on limited evidence. Clinical studies have shown that a starting dose of 400 mg/day is quite effective for GISTs containing a mutation in exon 11 of the *KIT* gene. Patients with exon 11 *KIT* mutations can delay taking higher doses until there is no more benefit from 400 mg/day, and this will likely give them the best quality of life as well as an optimal chance of disease control. Some other types of primary mutations in GISTs appear to be less responsive to imatinib than those in exon 11. Preliminary evidence suggests that some patients with GISTs harboring a mutation in exon 9 of the KIT gene might benefit from using higher starting doses of imatinib, such as 600 mg/day or even 800 mg/day. Few data exist on

The optimal dose of a cancer drug is generally a compromise between the benefits of higher amounts of the drug to stop your tumors versus the increased risks for adverse side effects at these higher doses.

patients who take more than 800 mg/day. If at some point your tumor is becoming resistant to lower doses of imatinib, then your dose may be increased or the drug therapy changed to sunitinib (see Question 82).

The 400 or 600 mg doses of imatinib are generally taken once daily, although some patients prefer to split the doses by taking the smaller (100 mg) size pills. If 800 mg are prescribed, then you should take 400 mg twice a day. Some oncologists recommend dividing any dose in half and taking it twice daily to minimize nausea or other unpleasant side effects. If you have any serious problems with the function of your liver, your physician may choose to start at a dose lower than 400 mg/day.

The starting dose of sunitinib is usually 50 mg daily for 4 weeks followed by 2 weeks off of the drug, called the "washout" period. This allows the patient's body to recover from any side effects of the drug. Some patients have expressed concerns about whether their tumors might "wake up" to some extent when they are off of the drug for 2 weeks. Recent clinical studies have investigated whether patients would benefit from taking sunitinib at a somewhat lower daily dose of 37.5 mg continuously each day without the washout period. The results of these trials should become available soon.

In the case of targeted therapy (imatinib and sunitinib), specific blood tests must be taken before you start therapy and while you are on it.

Imatinib is manufactured in 100 and 400 mg tablets; thus, your physician can change your dose based on your test results and symptoms. Sunitinib is manufactured in 12.5, 25, and 50 mg capsules for the same reason.

If your primary care provider prescribes a new medication, notify the physician who is prescribing the imatinib or the sunitinib. Adjustments to your dose may be needed if you are taking certain other medications that interfere with your body's normal processing of imatinib and sunitinib (see Question 62 and Tables 4 and 5 for a list of the medications that either increase or decrease levels of imatinib and sunitinib).

60. Why do I need routine blood tests during the time I am taking targeted cancer therapy?

Routine blood tests are common while taking certain medications, even those that are not meant to treat cancer. In the case of targeted therapy (imatinib and sunitinib), specific blood tests must be taken before you start therapy and while you are on it.

Just like the routine monitoring of the tumor helps your physician know whether your condition is improving or worsening, blood tests during imatinib and sunitinib therapy will help the physician develop your ongoing treatment plan. Based on the test results, your physician may change doses, give new medications, or suspend or stop therapy completely. These tests also assist in the diagnosis of certain adverse, sometimes life-threatening conditions that can result from the therapy.

Before beginning therapy with either imatinib or sunitinib, you will have a **complete blood count**, which measures the number, type, and/or size of red blood cells, **white blood cells**, and **platelets**. These first test results are important because as your treatment with the targeted cell therapy continues your blood test results will be compared with the beginning values. While taking imatinib or sunitinib, you may develop **anemia**, which can cause significant fatigue and may also suggest that you have internal bleeding. If your white cell count becomes very low, you may become susceptible to infection (see Question 61). If the number of your platelets decreases, you may develop bruising under the skin and bleeding, which can eventually lead to anemia.

In addition to the complete blood count, your physician will probably order a **metabolic panel**, which surveys certain substances in your blood so that the physician can determine whether your kidneys and liver are functioning normally.

Complete blood count

A blood test that measures the number, type, and/or size of red blood cells, white blood cells, and platelets.

White blood cells

Blood cells that protect the body from infection or disease.

Platelets

Found in blood; assists in clotting of blood.

Anemia

A low level of red blood cells, which carry oxygen in the blood.

Metabolic panel

Tests of certain substances in blood that determine whether the kidneys and liver are functioning normally; tests include but are not limited to the following: blood urea nitrogen, creatinine, total protein, albumin, bilirubin, AST, ALT, and alkaline phosphatase.

While you are taking imatinib, blood tests are normally done at each visit to your oncologist. Some oncologists recommend more frequent testing in the early weeks and months of new therapy. After being on imatinib for a while, blood work will generally be done every 1 to 2 months. When you are taking sunitinib, blood tests should be repeated before each 4-week cycle of therapy. Having blood tests regularly will help the physician to recognize subtle changes in your blood, thus ensuring that the treatment is not harming you.

61. What precautions do I need to take if my white blood counts are low? Can I do anything to boost my red blood cell and white blood cell counts?

Frequent complete blood counts are done to determine whether your white cell count has dropped to levels that may require further evaluation for additional precautions and medication adjustment. **Neutropenia** occurs when **neutrophils,** certain types of white cells, reach low levels. High levels of white cells, called **neutrophilia,** usually indicate that your body is fighting an acute infection. Conversely, when you have neutropenia, you may not have enough white cells to fight infection. Neutropenia is a potential side effect of some medications, including imatinib and sunitinib.

If you have a low level of white cells, you will need to avoid crowds and people with known infections. If you do get sick, having a low white cell count makes it more difficult for you to fight infection. Extremely low white counts may require you to stop therapy because of the risk of developing of a life-threatening infection.

Always consider your lifestyle when you are being treated for cancer. You must practice a healthy lifestyle when you are more susceptible to infection: Eat a well-balanced diet, and get a good night's sleep. Manage your stress, and exercise after consultation with your physician.

Neutropenia

Low level of white blood cells.

Neutrophil

White blood cell that destroys microorganisms and fights infection.

Neutrophilia

An increase in the number of neutrophils in the blood.

A special medication (such as Neulasta™ [pegfilgrastim]) may be used to help your body make more white blood cells. These drugs are commonly used in patients who are receiving conventional chemotherapy, but occasionally, they are needed in patients who are taking targeted cancer therapy.

Red blood cells use **hemoglobin** to carry oxygen to your body tissues. Anemia occurs when your red cell count gets too low. Low red cell counts can mean that you are bleeding internally, and your physician will look for the source of the bleeding. You may also have **iron-deficiency anemia**, which can cause fatigue and sometimes shortness of breath and can be treated with iron-rich foods. An iron supplement can cause constipation and stomach upset. Thus, your physician may choose not to prescribe it, especially if you already have nausea, vomiting, or heartburn. Your physician may consider prescribing epoetin alfa (Procrit™), which helps to build the number of red blood cells. Increasing your red blood cell count can make you feel less tired and stronger.

Hemoglobin

The oxygen-carrying component of red blood cells.

Iron-deficiency anemia

Anemia caused by lack of iron in the diet or from chronic bleeding.

62. What are the most common side effects from imatinib or sunitinib?

The adverse side effects of both imatinib and sunitinib are generally much more moderate than those of traditional types of chemotherapy. The severity of a drug's adverse side effect is generally ranked by oncology researchers on a scale of 1 through 5. Grade 1 is the mildest, and grade 5 is death. The side effects reported for imatinib and sunitinib are much more frequently grades 1 or 2 (less severe), although a few patients do experience grade 3 or grade 4 reactions.

The adverse side effects of both imatinib and sunitinib are generally much more moderate than those of traditional types of chemotherapy.

Most of the side effects associated with imatinib and sunitinib appear within the first few months of starting therapy. Typically, they are relatively easy to manage while still taking the drug. Many side effects are dose related and may diminish if your dose is decreased. Patients frequently report that their side effects with imatinib lessen the longer they have been on the drug. You and your physician can decide which side effects are tolerable and which are not. Your optimal drug dose prevents tumor progression with a minimal number of side effects.

Imatinib Side Effects

The most common side effects that clinical trial patients report include anemia, edema, fatigue, fever, muscle aches/cramps, diarrhea, gastrointestinal cramping/nausea, swollen eyes, and skin rash. The frequency and severity of imatinib's side effects are dose dependent, with more grades 3 and 4 adverse events associated with the higher 800 mg/day dose than the 400 mg/day dose. Table 4 describes the clinical uses, contraindications, side effects, serious adverse reactions, and special considerations for imatinib.

A more common side effect of imatinib, **edema,** can occur in your feet, hands, and most commonly around your eyes. Although puffiness around your eyes can be disturbing, it is not a threat to your vision. If you begin to retain fluid in your lungs, heart, or abdomen, the problem is more serious; you should contact your physician. If you start to accumulate fluid around your lungs (**pleural effusion**) or in your abdomen (**ascites**), then you may need a **diuretic,** which relieves the fluid retention by allowing your body to produce more urine.

Muscle cramps are common and are often treated with calcium and magnesium supplements. Although quinine is not approved for leg cramps, it may be prescribed if your nighttime leg cramps are severe. Skin rashes, especially itchy ones, can be annoying but are usually not life threatening. Most likely, an oral antihistamine and/or a steroid cream can be applied directly to the rash.

Although bone, muscle, joint pain, and abdominal pain are not common, you should notify your physician if these occur. Taking other medications with your cancer therapy (includ-

Edema

Excessive accumulation of fluid.

Pleural effusion

Fluid in the lungs.

Ascites

The accumulation of fluid in the abdomen.

Diuretic

A medication used to treat the accumulation of too much fluid in the body (edema); assists in the discharge of the fluid through urine.

ing over the counter drugs) calls for caution. Your doctor can make recommendations about the pain medications that he or she feels are safe for you to use with imatinib.

The toxic effects of imatinib on the liver may cause a few patients to develop more serious problems with their liver function. Uncommonly, these liver toxicities become severe enough to require some kind of intervention—usually a temporary interruption of the drug dosing until liver function improves (see Question 65).

Bleeding can occur in many sites, including from the tumors as they respond to the drug therapy. Bleeding may also develop in the conjunctiva of the eye (red eye), nose, urine, gastrointestinal tract, and brain and under the skin. Most bleeding is not life threatening, although bleeding from the gastrointestinal tract or tumor can be serious and is considered an emergency.

Sunitinib Side Effects

Sunitinib is not as well tolerated as imatinib, but the side effects are manageable for most people without dose reductions. Common side effects include fatigue, diarrhea, gastrointestinal discomfort, **hypertension**, skin disorders, muscle pain, anemia, and low white blood cell counts. Table 5 describes the clinical uses, contraindications, side effects, serious adverse reactions, and special considerations for sunitinib.

Sunitinib blocks the formation of new blood vessels, resulting in side effects that are also observed for other drugs of this class. Sunitinib can cause hypertension in patients. Having physical exams and monitoring your blood pressure and blood counts are important while taking sunitinib. Blood pressure medications can be used to reduce the hypertension that sunitinib may cause. In the case of severely high blood pressure, therapy may be temporarily stopped.

Hypertension

Abnormally high arterial blood pressure that is usually indicated by an adult systolic blood pressure of 140 mm Hg or greater or a diastolic blood pressure of 90 mm Hg or greater.

Table 4 Imatinib (Gleevec™)

Generic Name (Trade Name) [Pharmaceutical Manufactuer] How Supplied	Clinical Uses	Contradictions	Most Common Side Effects and Adverse Reactions
Imatinib mesylate (Gleevec™) [Novartis] 100 mg and 400 mg tablets to be taken daily by mouth Starting dosage is usually 400 mg	*Treatment of Kit (CD117) positive inoperable and/or metastatic malignant GIST *Treatment of CML (Chronic myeloid leukemia)	Hypersensitvity to imatinib or any of the components of Gleevec	Nausea Vomiting Fluid retention (sometimes severe) Muscle cramps Skin rash Diarrhea Heartburn Headache Serious Adverse Reactions (Report these immediately to your physician): Difficulty breathing Severe fluid retention Liver problems (such as jaundice) Potential for bleeding, especially in the elderly

(continues)

Table 4   (continued)

Special Considerations	
Safety in children under 18years has not been established.	Capsules are usually taken daily with meals and a large glass of water
Side effects, especially edema, and adverse reactions can be dose related. Decreasing the dosage may decrease side effects.	A complete blood count and liver function tests are usually taken before initiating therapy and thereafter to monitor for abnormal white cell counts and abnormal liver function.
The following medications may increase the levels of imatinib in your blood: *ketoconazole (Nizoral) *itraconazole (Sporanox) *erythromycin (Many different names) *clarithromycin (Biaxin)	It is advisable to monitor your weight in case you develop sudden weight gain that might be excessive fluid retention.
The following medications may reduce the levels of imatinib in your blood: *dexamethasone (a steroid medication) *phenytoin (Dilantin) *carbamazepine (Tegretol and others) *rifampicin (Rifadin and others) *phenobarbital (Luminal and others) *St. John's wort (over the counter herbal supplement)	Because imatinib can cause severe birth defects and the increased potential for miscarriage, women of childbearing age should not become pregnant while taking imatinib. Men should also use birth control if their partners can become pregnant.
	Mothers should not breastfeed while taking imatinib.
	For patients unable to swallow tablets, the tablets may be dissolved in water or apple juice. To be consumed immediately after dissolving.

Table 5 Sunitinib (Sutent™)

Generic Name (Trade Name) [Pharmaceutical Manufactuer] How Supplied	Clinical Uses	Contradictions	Most Common Side Effects and Adverse Reactions
Sunitinib malate (Sutent™) [Pfizer] 12.5 mg, 25 mg, 50 mg capsules Starting dosage is 50 mg daily by mouth for 4 weeks followed by 2 weeks off	Treatment of GI stromal tumors that are resistant to imatinib Treatment of GI stromal tumors in patients who are unable to tolerate imatinib Advanced kidney cancer	Hypersensitvity to sunitinib or any of its components Special caution: Patients with cardiovascular conditions such as prior myocardial infarction, unstable angina, coronary artery bypass graft, congestive heart failure, stroke or transient ischemic attack, or pulmonary embolism require special cardiac monitoring, particularly left ventricular ejection fraction evaluation (see Special Considerations) St. John's wort may not be taken during sunitinib therapy	Fatigue Diarrhea Nausea Mouth irritation Heartburn Altered taste Rash Skin Dryness Vomiting Constipation Skin and hair discoloration Anorexia Nosebleed Serious Adverse Reactions: Hemorrhage (primarily at tumor site) Congestive heart failure High blood pressure

(continues)

Table 5   (continued)

Special Considerations	
Safety in children under 18 years has not been established.	Sunitinib should be discontinued in patients who develop congestive heart failure (CHF). Doses should be interrupted or reduced in patients without clinical signs and symptoms of CHF but with an ejection fraction of <50% and >20% below baseline.
Tests for adrenal insufficiency should be taken in patients experiencing stress such as surgery, trauma, or severe infection.	
Capsules may be taken with or without food.	Difficulty breathing, bleeding, and bruising should be reported immediately to a physician. They can be signs of life-threatening events.
A complete blood count and blood chemistries are usually taken before initiating therapy in each cycle.	High blood pressure, although potentially serious, can be treated with standard anti-hypertensive therapies.
Women of childbearing age should not become pregnant or breastfeed while on sunitinib therapy.	GI side effects can be treated with anti-nausea and anti-diarrheal medications.
Dose reduction should be considered if prescribed ketoconazole (Nizoral™, an antifungal medication) during sunitinib therapy.	
Dose increase should be considered if prescribed rifampin (Rifadin™, Rimactane™, an antibiotic) during sunitinib therapy.	

Table 6 Management of side effects of imatinib and sunitinib

Side effect	Management suggestions
Nausea	Take with meals; divide dosage to take twice daily; take with full glass of water; if severe, physician may prescribe Phenergan™, Zofran™ or other anti-nausea/emetic medication; light diet with foods such mashed potatoes, cola drinks, ginger ale
Vomiting	Same management as nausea
Fluid retention	Weigh yourself daily; physician should evaluate for treatment with diuretics. If treated with diuretics, be aware of side effects, many of which are the same as those in this table.
Muscle cramps	Take calcium and magnesium supplements.
Muscle aches and pains	No aspirin, no Tylenol™ unless approved by physician; it is okay to take ibuprofen (Advil™ or Motrin IB™) or naproxyn (Aleve™); be careful about the use of over-the-counter pain medications
Skin rash and peeling, dryness, thickness or cracking of skin, blisters on hands and feet	Moisturizers, over-the-counter cortisone cream may help but may require prescription-strength cream or ointment; itchy rashes may improve with diphenhydramine (Benadryl™) or other antihistamines
Diarrhea and GI cramps	Over-the-counter anti-diarrheal agents (do not take ones containing aspirin); try BRAT diet (bananas, rice, applesauce, toast)
Heartburn	Take with meals; remain upright for at least 1 hour after taking medication; sometimes Protonix™ or other acid-reducers are prescribed. Over-the-counter antacids such as Tums™, Rolaids™ may help.
Headache	Do not take Tylenol™ unless approved by physician. Ibuprofen (Advil™, Motrin IB™ Aleve™) may help; no aspirin; massage forehead temples
High blood pressure	Physician should evaluate for treatment with anti-hypertensives.
Fatigue	Physician should evaluate for hypothyroidism and anemia; if fatigue is a result of insomnia, sleeplessness, or depression, still be evaluated for medication

(continues)

Table 6 (continued)

Side effect	Management suggestions
Anemia	Physician should evaluate for bleeding source; iron-rich foods; iron supplementation; evaluation for Procrit™
	Avoid crowds and sick people; keep your skin moisturized, particularly your feet (where circulation tends to be poor.
Neutropenia (low white cell counts)	If you develop fever, do not take fever-reducing medication until you are evaluated for the source of the fever; evaluation for medications like Neulasta™
Loss of hair pigmentation	May not respond to hair dye
Skin discoloration	Usually results from the color of the tablets and capsules; however, jaundice must be evaluated for liver involvement
Intestinal gas (flatulence)	Avoid gas-producing foods such as cauliflower, large helpings of beans, broccoli
Fever	Do not take fever-reducing medications until you are evaluated for the source of the fever

Some concern has existed in the past about patients who have **cardiovascular** problems and require sunitinib. A physician's careful monitoring is very important if you have existing heart problems, such as a prior heart attack, **angina**, stroke, or **congestive heart failure**. Sunitinib may have a negative effect on the left ventricle of the heart and may eventually cause congestive heart failure. Congestive heart failure can become life threatening because your heart is not able to pump adequately. If you experience fluid retention, cough, and difficulty breathing while on sunitinib, contact your physician.

Many patients on sunitinib complain of fatigue. In some patients, fatigue is associated with hypothyroidism that the sunitinib therapy causes. The energy level improves if the patients are treated with thyroid hormone replacement.

Sunitinib, as well as other anti-angiogenesis drugs, can cause a painful hand-foot syndrome that is characterized by tender and blistered skin in these areas. The orange-brown color of the sunitinib compound may produce a skin discoloration that should not be confused with **jaundice**, a condition that results from too much **bilirubin**. Jaundice can indicate severe liver disease or inflammation and should be evaluated by a physician.

Bleeding can be an adverse reaction to sunitinib. The most common site for bleeding is your nose. As with imatinib, gastrointestinal bleeding requires immediate evaluation. Coughing up blood can be a sign of bleeding from the lung and is considered a medical emergency. A number of common side effects and suggestions for management are listed in Table 6.

63. What about long-term side effects of imatinib and sunitinib?

Because imatinib has only been approved by the FDA for use in GIST patients since 2002 and sunitinib since 2006, only very limited long-term safety data are available for these drugs. We can't currently rule out the possibility of unforeseen side effects for a patient who has used the drug continuously for many years or decades. Furthermore, subtle or very rare side effects may go unnoticed during the first clinical studies.

Adverse reactions found from animal studies are also sometimes difficult to put into perspective. These animals may suffer from certain adverse reactions to a drug when humans don't. For instance, laboratory rats receiving imatinib have higher rates of **urogenital** tract tumors. We don't yet know whether this will happen to patients. Human tumors are slow to develop, and very few patients have been on the drug for more than 5 years.

The Food and Drug Administration (FDA) and the manufacturer of the drug will take any reports of new side effects seriously and will investigate them further. Sometimes more clinical studies are needed to learn about a new side effect. If more data substantiate the preliminary report, then the drug's package insert and its prescribing information for physicians will be amended to document the newly recognized side effect.

In recent months, scientific reports have described two previously unrecognized side effects of imatinib. One study noted bone mineralization problems and low vitamin D levels with longer use. Another study described cardiac heart failure after the start of imatinib for a small number of leukemia patients who mostly had pre-existing risk factors for heart problems.

Do not panic if you hear a news report about potential new side effects of a drug. Discuss any new information with your doctor.

Because imatinib has only been approved since 2002 and sunitinib since 2006, no long-term safety data are available for these drugs.

Urogenital
Related to the urinary excretion or reproductive systems.

Medical Therapy of Metastatic GIST

64. Can other drugs, foods, or supplements interfere with targeted cancer therapy?

Yes, other substances can interfere with your targeted therapy. Before prescribing targeted cancer therapy, your physician should always be aware of any drugs or supplements that you are taking. Also, be honest about your alcohol consumption.

Grapefruit juice should be avoided during your therapy, and alcohol should be consumed in a moderate amount (generally, one alcoholic drink per day for women and two for men). Although no other specific foods or beverages interfere with your drug therapy, you must follow a balanced diet or a diet that your nutritionist designed.

Certain drugs may require that your dose be adjusted up or down, depending on the drug.

The following medications may **increase** the levels of imatinib in your blood: ketoconazole (Nizoral™), itraconazole (Sporanox™), erythromycin (manufactured under many different names), and clarithromycin (Biaxin™). The following medications may **reduce** the levels of imatinib in your blood: dexamethasone (a steroid medication), phenytoin (Dilantin™), carbamazepine (Tegretol™ and others), rifampicin (Rifadin™ and others), and phenobarbital (Luminal™ and others).

Tylenol™ should be used sparingly because its combination with imatinib may lead to liver failure.

If you are taking a blood thinner medication (such as warfarin, also known as Coumadin™), the dose of that medication may need adjustment because imatinib can change its concentration. Check with your physician about this as well as birth control pills, which may interact with the drug.

Many patients think that they need to inform their physicians of only their routine prescription medications; however,

Describes medications, herbs, or supplements that can be purchased without a prescription.

over-the-counter medications and dietary supplements are also important. Because St. John's wort has a negative effect on both imatinib and sunitinib, do not continue to take it while you are taking either of the targeted therapies. If you are taking it for depression, ask your physician for an appropriate substitute.

65. What is drug-induced liver toxicity, and is there anything I can do for it?

Many drugs, including imatinib and sunitinib, are broken down through the liver. Sometimes when your liver doesn't process the drugs fast or effectively enough, the byproducts of drugs or the drugs themselves can cause your liver to become toxic, which means that it could fail to work. This is an extremely rare side effect of targeted therapy. Because your physician routinely monitors liver function, abnormal results or certain changes in the test results will require reassessment of your dose. Decreasing the dose or interrupting targeted therapy for even 1 week can improve liver function. Because Tylenol™ is also metabolized in the liver, its use should be discontinued while you are using imatinib or sunitinib. Heavy alcohol consumption can also lead to a poorly functioning liver.

Physicians sometimes prescribe an oral steroid if targeted therapy is severely affecting the liver. Most patients are able to resume their targeted therapy after their liver function returns to normal. A recent study showed that treatment with steroids helped leukemia patients to resume therapy with imatinib after having persistent liver function problems that otherwise could not be resolved by temporarily stopping imatinib dosing.

66. How can a CT scan or an MRI determine a tumor's response to a cancer drug? What are stable disease, partial remission, and complete remission?

Radiologists evaluate GISTs and measure them generally in two or possibly three dimensions. Those measurements are then compared with a baseline CT scan or MRI and scans obtained later while on therapy.

Several other methods are used to measure response to therapy on radiologic tests. No optimal method has been widely adopted. The major deficit of conventional systems is that they mostly measure tumor size. Tumor size tells only part of the story, as a response to therapy in some patients can just change the consistency of the tumor without shrinking it (see Question 68).

A complete response to therapy, where the cancer disappears completely on the radiologic studies, is the best. This rarely happens. A partial response means a reduction in the volume of cancer by 50% or more. Stable disease implies that the tumor did not grow in size or grew or shrank less than 25%. Although the cancer will hopefully shrink, preventing it from growing further is also beneficial. An increase in tumor size of more than 25% represents progression of disease. This is a reason to stop the current treatment or alter the dose.

67. When are PET scans useful in a patient who is taking targeted cancer therapy? What is a PET flare?

A PET scan tracks the uptake of a radioactive sugar within the body after it has been injected into a patient's vein. How much sugar a specific tissue uses is a measure of its energy **metabolism** and its potential for growth. Because cancer cells are growing rapidly, they will often have a different level

Metabolism

The breaking down of substances in the body to generate energy.

of metabolism than the surrounding normal tissues. Thus, a PET scan makes a distinction between diseased and normal tissues.

Whereas a PET scan measures sugar metabolism, a CT scan detects the actual physical structures of the body by showing how X-ray energy passes through the different types of tissues. A CT scan does not give any information about the metabolism of tissues. If something happens to speed up or slow down the sugar metabolism of a specific tissue, then the result will be observed as changes in PET activity. If the process did not alter the actual structure of this tissue, then the CT scan would remain unchanged.

A PET scan detects potentially cancerous tissue as a "hot spot" (Figure 8). A PET scan cannot directly demonstrate that a hot area is actually caused by cancer cells versus other non-cancerous conditions (such as inflammation). Your doctor can decide whether a certain hot area on a PET scan is cancer. In general, PET scans are not required very often in GISTs. They are primarily used for research purposes. In some patients,

Whereas a PET scan measures sugar metabolism, a CT scan detects the actual physical structures of the body by showing how X-ray energy passes through the different types of tissues.

Before   After

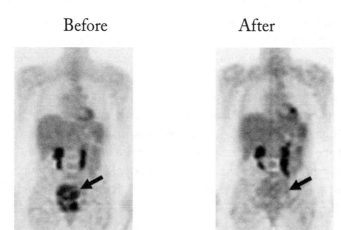

Figure 8   Radiographic response to imatinib. PET scans are shown prior to and after imatinib.

PET imaging may be needed to show whether a targeted cancer therapy drug has succeeded early during the treatment course. Physical changes in the tumor, such as shrinkage, take longer to become evident on a CT scan. A PET scan might be needed if the results from a CT scan are unclear.

A PET flare, or an increase in metabolic activity of a tumor, during drug therapy may indicate that a tumor is no longer responding to the drug even before the tumor has grown enough to appear different on a CT scan. A PET scan alone, however, does not substitute for a CT scan's information. If a patient stops taking targeted cancer therapy, then within a brief period he or she may experience a PET flare. Inactive GIST cells remaining in the patient's body can "reawaken" if the drug therapy is withdrawn. Overall tumor growth may follow shortly unless the drug treatment is resumed.

68. What about CT scans for patients who are taking targeted cancer therapy?

CT scans are still the pre-ferred way to monitor GISTs routinely dur-ing treatment; however, the size measure-ments on a CT scan do not always reflect how much a tu-mor is respond-ing to targeted cancer therapy.

CT scans are still the preferred way to monitor GISTs routinely during treatment; however, the size measurements on a CT scan do not always reflect how much a tumor is responding to targeted cancer therapy. Patients and their doctors need to evaluate the overall characteristics of the lesions, looking for signs that the tumors have undergone a cystic transformation. Generally, the cystic area that develops as a tumor dies has a dark, uniform appearance, with distinct smooth edges separating it from adjacent normal tissue, as if it were a simple "hole" (Figure 9). A living solid tumor has a more irregular appearance of varying shades of lightness and darkness within it, typically with a fuzzy bright white halo around its outside edge. An initial increase in the overall size of a tumor on CT does not always mean that the cancer treated with target therapy is still growing. As GIST cells die, they break open and can spill their contents into their surroundings; this may cause fluid swelling of the residual lesion, which may be mis-interpreted as tumor growth.

Pre-treatment   6 months   10 months

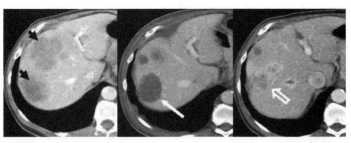

Figure 9   Response and resistance to imatinib. Serial CT scans of the liver are shown. The patient had multiple liver metastases (arrowheads) and had a response to imatinib at 6 months. Note the darker gray appearance which means less uptake of intravenous contrast. The presence of a small nodule (solid arrow) represents residual tumor. After another 4 months on imatinib, the patient progressed and developed a large tumor (open arrow) in the liver. From Van der Zwan SM, DeMatteo RP. Gastrointestinal stromal tumor: 5 years later. Cancer. 2005 Nov 1;104(9):1781–8.

Tumors that start to grow again after a good drug response may develop a solid mass that originates at the outer rim of the cystic spot. Sometimes the new solid mass grows inward into the liquefied zone of the cyst rather than growing outward into the adjacent normal tissue. If the new mass grows inward, then there may not be an increase in the overall dimensions of the GIST lesion, even though the tumor is once again progressing. This inward growth pattern is called a "nodule within a mass" or a "nodule within a nodule." When a nodule within a mass happens, the inside area of the lesion will no longer look consistent as a plain dark area but instead will have signs of a solid mass inside (Figure 9). Your radiologist will look for any signs of a nodule within a mass during your routine follow-up CT scans while you remain on targeted cancer therapy.

69. Does the degree of tumor shrinkage from targeted cancer therapy provide any indication about my long-term prognosis? What is tumor progression?

Patients see tumor shrinkage as a sign that their drug therapy is working. Clinical studies show that the maximum amount of tumor shrinkage in response to imatinib or sunitinib does not predict how long you will receive benefit from these drugs. The most important thing is that the drug halts any further growth of your tumors. Patients in clinical studies who had stabilized tumors without much shrinkage fared just as well overall as the patients who had significant shrinkage. Patients who did not achieve stability in their tumors did not do as well. Their disease showed **tumor progression**, which means the tumors continued to grow larger.

Although you may be pleased if your tumors remain stable or shrink on imatinib, your long-term prognosis cannot be predicted. GISTs and their management are complex and are not like other cancers. Predicting your long-term prognosis based on your initial response to targeted therapy is not entirely reliable.

70. Why should I comply with my doctor's prescription for oral cancer drugs?

Targeted cancer therapy should be taken exactly as your doctor directs. You should practice **persistency**, meaning that you should take your cancer drug on an uninterrupted basis for the entire duration of the therapy. Patients who opt on their own to stop taking their cancer drugs for various reasons, including having uncomfortable side effects or forgetting to refill the prescription, may have rapid disease progression.

You must also adhere to the exact specified dose. Do not change your dose on your own. A smaller dose than your doctor has prescribed may lack full effectiveness against your

Tumor progression

Enlarging or spreading of the tumor.

Persistency

Taking drug on an uninterrupted basis for the entire duration of the therapy.

Patients who stop taking their cancer drugs for various reasons, including having uncomfortable side effects or forgetting to refill the prescription, may have rapid disease progression.

tumors, whereas a higher one may cause too many **toxicities**. If you accidentally forget to take your drug on a single day, simply resume your normal dose the next day.

A recent survey showed that many patients need to do a better job of complying with their doctor's directions for dosing. About 30% of patients did not take their therapy for at least 30 consecutive days in the first year. Using a weekly pill-box organizer or establishing a routine time of day to take your therapy can help you to stay on schedule. Also, anticipate when your prescription needs to be refilled, and mark the date on your calendar to avoid running out of pills at home.

Toxicities
Undesirable side effects from medications.

71. Can I take birth control pills while I am using targeted therapy drugs? What risks do these drugs pose if I become pregnant?

The FDA assigns risk categories to drugs. Because imatinib and sunitinib can potentially harm a fetus, they have been assigned the risk category of "D," meaning that a positive evidence of fetal risk exists. Nevertheless, potential benefits from the drug outweigh the risk. For example, the drug may be acceptable in a life-threatening situation or serious disease if safe drugs can't be used or are ineffective.

Women of childbearing potential who have GISTs should consider two scenarios. Nonpregnant patients should avoid pregnancy, and an effective method of birth control should be used. Birth control pills should not be used as the sole method of birth control while you are on targeted therapy. Although condoms and diaphragms are considered reliable, a combination of methods may be the most dependable. Abstinence and more permanent methods (such as tubal ligation in women and vasectomy in men) are also options. In patients who become pregnant, a decision may need to be made between stopping the drug and risking allowing your tumor to grow, terminating the pregnancy, or going forward with both the

Medical Therapy of Metastatic GIST

pregnancy and drug, realizing that you could deliver a baby with serious birth defects.

If you are a female partner of a male who is being treated with either imatinib or sunitinib, you should also use birth control. Do not breastfeed while on imatinib or sunitinib. Data clearly show that imatinib is excreted in human milk; although fewer data are available on sunitinib, breastfeeding is still not recommended.

72. Is the treatment of children with GISTs the same as that of adults?

Very few cases of GIST in children have been reported in the world. Some statistics suggest, however, that most children with GISTs are older than 10 years, are female, and have primary tumors mostly in the stomach. Most children do not have either a *KIT* or *PDGFRA* gene mutation. Like adults, surgery is recommended if the GIST is operable. Unlike adults, however, multiple primary tumors often are present. GISTs in children tend to grow more slowly than in adults. Metastatic GIST in children spreads not only to the liver and peritoneum (as in adults) but also to the nearby lymph nodes, an extremely rare metastatic location in adults.

Imatinib benefits up to 85% of adults with metastatic or un-resectable primary GISTs. Unfortunately, imatinib seems to be less effective in children than in most adults. Children may respond better to sunitinib. The lack of data about children with GIST can be frustrating to parents and clinicians alike. Currently, a multicenter study is researching patients with GIST who are under 30 years old. Because pediatric GISTs are so rare, parents are advised to seek out a pediatric sarcoma specialist. Advances in our understanding of cancer are moving quickly, and seeking treatment at a sarcoma research center will allow the families and parents to be close to the latest breaking news and to tap into the latest findings and perhaps promising investigational trials.

73. What other treatment options are available besides molecular therapy? Are future treatments for GISTs on the horizon?

The standard of care for almost all patients with metastatic GIST is targeted molecular therapy. In certain circumstances, your doctor may want to add another type of treatment, including surgery or **tumor ablation**, which is discussed in the following questions. Although imatinib and sunitinib represent major advances in GIST therapy, researchers are studying other compounds to determine whether they will work after these two drugs fail (see Questions 85–88).

The standard of care for almost all patients with metastatic GISTs is targeted molecular therapy.

74. Is surgery useful for metastatic GISTs? If the disease is confined to my liver, can I get a transplant?

A number of centers in the world have now investigated the issue of whether surgery is useful for metastatic GIST, but a proper scientific clinical trial has not been conducted. From the collective experience of these centers, surgery appears to have little value in patients who have multiple tumors that have become resistant to imatinib or sunitinib. Meanwhile, in patients with stable disease or a single site of resistance, surgery may be helpful. Some doctors suspect that getting rid of all visible disease will prolong the time to development of widespread resistance to medical therapy. Discuss with your doctor the options for surgical resection of your metastatic GIST.

In other patients, partial removal of tumor may alleviate symptoms from metastatic GIST. For example, if all your disease cannot be removed but you develop bleeding or intestinal obstruction from one particular tumor, then surgery may be useful.

Transplantation is not practiced for patients with metastatic GISTs to the liver. The risk of developing recurrent disease is

Tumor ablation

The destruction of a tumor without actually removing it.

quite high, even if the entire liver is removed. The medications that a patient must take after a liver transplant to prevent rejection of the new organ can promote growth of residual microscopic GIST that exists outside of the liver.

75. What are tumor ablation, hepatic artery embolization, radiofrequency ablation, and cryoablation?

Tumor ablation is the destruction of a tumor without actually removing it. In general, ablation is not as effective as surgical removal. Nevertheless, ablation can be useful in selected instances. In some cases, the entire tumor can be destroyed, especially if the tumor is small. With larger tumors, it is more likely that a small part of the tumor will survive and begin to grow again at some point. Several techniques of ablation are available, including **hepatic artery embolization, radiofrequency ablation (RFA),** and **cryotherapy**. Each method acts in a different way, as described below. Any of the various procedures can be repeated in the future if your tumor grows back. If you have multiple tumors or a large tumor, you may need to be treated a few times in the first month or two to cover all of your disease.

Hepatic artery embolization is the injection of particles into the hepatic artery in order to destroy GISTs that have spread to the liver. The particles can be thought of as microscopic sand that clogs the blood vessels feeding the tumor. A tumor's survival in the liver depends largely on blood that the hepatic artery supplies. Part of the hepatic artery can be clogged safely because your liver receives blood from another vessel called the **portal vein**. Many doctors use particles that also have a chemotherapy agent attached to them. It is unclear whether particles alone or particles with attached chemotherapy are better to use. Each group of doctors has their preference.

An **interventional radiologist,** who is specialized in performing invasive procedures under image guidance, performs he-

Hepatic artery embolization

The injection of particles into the hepatic artery in order to destroy a GIST that has spread to the liver.

Radiofrequency ablation

Technique of inserting a metal probe into the tumor and exposing it to extreme heat.

Cryotherapy

Technique of inserting a metal probe into the tumor and exposing it to extreme cold.

Portal vein

A vein entering the liver.

Interventional radiologist

A radiologist who uses image guidance to gain access to vessels and organs in order to treat conditions under the skin; uses catheters, balloons, and stents.

patic artery embolization. You usually come into the hospital on the day of the procedure. You will be lightly sedated. The procedure, which takes about 2 hours, is carried out while you are lying flat on a table. The skin in your leg (usually the right leg) is numbed. Then a small tube is placed into the main artery in your leg. An X-ray machine is used to monitor the location of the small tube, which is passed through a large artery called the **aorta** and then into the **hepatic artery**, which feeds your liver. The tube is advanced into either the right or left branch of the hepatic artery. From there, particles can be released. In general, it is desirable to selectively occlude the specific blood vessels that are supplying a tumor and preserve the vessels going to normal liver. At the end of the procedure, the small tube is removed from your leg. You will have to lie flat for 4 to 6 hours afterward to make sure that the wound heals and that you do not bleed.

Embolization can cause a number of side effects; thus, most patients are admitted to the hospital for 2 to 4 days. In general, the magnitude of the side effects is proportional to the amount of tumor that is destroyed. In other words, if you have a large tumor, a lot of side effects can be expected if it was completely embolized. The dead tissue that results from the embolization releases toxic substances into your bloodstream, thus making you sick. The most common side effect is nausea. Although this can be controlled with special medication, you may not wish to eat for a day or so. Pain can occur, and you will receive medication for relief. Rarely, embolization will cause a problem with your heart or kidney function. Another unusual complication, called an abscess, is the formation of an infection in the dead tumor tissue. For this you would be treated with antibiotics. In rare situations, a drain may be placed into the infection. Commonly, the tube may adversely affect the artery in your leg. Bleeding can occur at the puncture site and form a large bruise called a **hematoma**. Occasionally, a patient may require an operation to repair the blood vessel if it was damaged and a **pseudoaneurysm**, or abnormality of the blood vessel wall, resulted.

Aorta

The large main artery that comes from the left ventricle of the heart that carries oxygenated blood.

Hepatic artery

An artery that carries blood to the liver.

Hematoma

A break in a blood vessel causing swelling.

Pseudoaneurysm

An abnormal dilation of the arterial wall at a previous site of catheter entry.

RFA and cryotherapy are used to destroy a tumor by inserting a metal probe into the tumor and exposing it to extremes of temperature. RFA heats the tumor while cryotherapy freezes it. RFA and cryotherapy can generally be used only if you have a limited number of tumors (usually less than five or six) that are small to medium in size (less than 5 cm). Either procedure can be performed in a variety of ways. **Percutaneous** means through the skin. An interventional radiologist can place the probe percutaneously—in which case you will require sedation during the procedure. RFA and cryotherapy can also be performed via laparoscopy or during an open surgical operation. Both require general anesthesia. Laparoscopy involves several small incisions in your abdomen. Open **laparotomy** is performed through a cut in your belly. Your doctor will decide which access is best based on the number, size, and location of your tumors. For instance, not all liver tumors can be reached via the percutaneous approach. Not all tumors can be treated with RFA or cryotherapy. If a tumor is close to a main bile duct, these techniques may be too risky. Also, if a tumor is near a large blood vessel, RFA and cryotherapy may not be advisable.

Percutaneous

Through the skin.

Laparotomy

An incision into the abdomen.

76. Can radiation be used to treat GIST and what are its side effects?

Radiation therapy depends on the high energy of certain electromagnetic waves. These powerful radiation rays can be controlled and directed toward a cancer. The aim is obviously to kill cancer cells. The two main types of radiation waves are X-rays and gamma rays. They differ in production and power and have different applications to cancer. Radiation is delivered from outside of the body. It penetrates through the skin and is targeted to the tumor. This is called external beam radiation.

Although radiation is commonly used to treat many cancers, it has not been used in many patients with GIST; therefore, its benefits are unproven.

Although radiation is commonly used to treat many cancers, it has not been used in many patients with GIST; therefore, its benefits are unproven. Nevertheless, your doctor may want to use radiation in certain circumstances. For instance, if you had a tumor in your pelvis, your doctor may want to give you radiation because it is useful for certain other pelvic tumors. **Radiation oncologists** can prepare a three-dimensional computer model of your tumor and then target radiation therapy to it while minimizing the effect on the surrounding tissue.

The side effects of radiation therapy depend on which part of the body is being irradiated. You might get diarrhea if the radiation affects the lining of the bowels that are close to the field of radiation. Radiation also generally causes fatigue. Finally, patients might have reduced white blood cells, red blood cells, or platelets if the radiation affects their bone marrow.

Radiation oncologist

A doctor who specializes in using radiation to treat cancer.

PART TEN

If a GIST Becomes Resistant to Drug Therapy

What is a drug-resistant tumor?

How will I know whether I have
drug-resistant tumors?

How does a tumor become resistant to
targeted cancer therapy?

More . . .

77. What is a drug-resistant tumor?

A tumor is drug resistant if it grows despite ongoing treatment with a specific cancer drug. Imatinib is generally the first targeted therapy that GIST patients try. Two classes of resistance to imatinib exist. A tumor has primary resistance if it failed initially to stay the same size or shrink during the first 6 months of imatinib therapy or it grew again within 6 months of the first dose. Other tumors may be controlled by imatinib for years before the drug stops being effective. Tumors in this case have acquired drug resistance. The average time to develop acquired resistance to imatinib is 2 years.

The underlying mechanisms for primary versus acquired **resistance** to imatinib appear different. Fortunately, only a small percentage of GIST patients have primary resistance to imatinib. Patients with primary resistance most often are wild type for *KIT* and *PDGFRA* genes or else have an exon 9 *KIT* mutation.

Patients may be surprised if their disease starts to grow again after years of successful treatment. Acquired drug resistance can develop at any point because the targeted therapy does not entirely eliminate all traces of the disease, but rather, it stabilizes the disease over the long term. An ongoing tug of war exists between the traits for growth in those GIST cells remaining in the body versus the ability of the drug to stop them. Patients need long-term follow-up to monitor whether the drug continues to work.

78. How will I know whether I have drug-resistant tumors?

Patients generally undergo routine CT scans to check the status of their disease. As explained in Question 68, GISTs responding well to targeted therapy do not always shrink, but they almost always transform into something like a liquefied cyst. The radiologist will examine these cystic areas on your CT scans for any signs that solid masses have returned, which indicates disease progression. A relapsing solid mass typically starts at the outer rim of these cystic areas. The relapsing mass may then grow into the interior space of the cyst or else outward into adjacent healthy tissue. The radiologist will also look for the appearance of new solid tumors at previously uninvolved locations. Increased activity of a tumor on a PET scan is another indication of tumor progression.

Sometimes small, solid GISTs within the liver are hard to see on CT films. After few weeks of targeted therapy, these previously unrecognized areas of disease might take on a more noticeable appearance as they become cystic in response to therapy. The truly new areas of disease must be distinguished from small, solid tumors that were initially overlooked.

Patients may have symptoms if their disease progresses. Firmness of the liver, expanding girth, feelings of fullness, a persistent low-grade fever, pain, and gastrointestinal blockages are all signs. GIST cells do not release substances that are detectable in standard blood tests.

79. How does a tumor become resistant to targeted cancer therapy?

A targeted therapy might fail in three general ways:

- An insufficient amount of the drug is present inside of the cancer cells to treat them effectively. This can happen two ways. Proteins in the tumor cell can pump the drug back out of the cell. If the tumor increases the number of pumps, then the drug gets removed from the cell before it has a chance to act. The other way is if the tumor finds a way to increase the protein that is causing the cancer to such high levels that it simply overwhelms the actions of the drug.
- The drug can no longer bind to its target protein. First consider this expression: "You can't force a square-peg into a round-hole." Imatinib represents the square-peg.

Doctors believe that these more mutated cells already existed at low levels within the tumors before therapy ever began.

Sunitinib may work after imatinib fails for two reasons: It can block other mutant forms of KIT not treatable by imatinib, and it has an additional mode of action by blocking the formation of new blood vessels within the tumors.

Secondary mutations

A second distinct mutation in the *KIT* or *PDGFRA* genes arising in addition to the primary mutation; a major cause of acquired resistance to drug therapy.

Imatinib fits precisely into a specific square-hole on the surface of abnormal KIT protein. When the square-peg imatinib docks into this particular square-hole on the KIT protein, it blocks the signals coming from KIT that instruct the GIST cells to grow. If the KIT protein acquires yet another mutation in addition to whatever mutation it had in the first place, then it now has two separate defects within its structure. The combination of these two defects may alter the shape of the KIT protein to where imatinib can no longer fit well. Thus, the KIT protein has acquired round-hole traits that are not compatible with square-peg imatinib. Doctors believe that these more mutated cells already existed at low levels within the tumors before therapy ever began.

• Sometimes, even as a drug successfully blocks cancer-causing signals from an abnormal protein, the cancer foils the drug by using alternative methods to signal for continued growth. Here is an analogy: The drug has successfully locked the front door on the cancer growth, but the cancer has found a way in through the back door. In this case, the signals for the cancer to grow have become re-routed through other proteins that are not targeted by the drug. Sometimes these alternate proteins also contain mutations that make them abnormal too.

80. What are strategies are used to overcome imatinib drug resistance?

Sunitinib was approved in 2006 as an effective drug for patients who are resistant to or cannot tolerate imatinib. Sunitinib may work after imatinib fails for two reasons: It can block other mutant forms of KIT not treatable by imatinib, and it has an additional mode of action by blocking the formation of new blood vessels within the tumors.

About half of the time, new mutations (called **secondary mutations**) in the *KIT* gene cause resistance to imatinib.

Reconsider our analogy about a square-peg not fitting well into a round-hole. Sunitinib has a different shape and different chemical characteristics than imatinib. Imagine sunitinib as a round-peg and imatinib as a square-peg. Over time, the KIT protein can become increasingly defective by acquiring more mutations. The shape of these more highly mutated KIT proteins harboring two or more distinct mutations may no longer be compatible with imatinib (square-peg); however, some of these abnormal forms of KIT might accommodate the properties of sunitinib (round-peg). Thus, sunitinib can block alternative mutant forms of KIT that imatinib cannot. Moreover, in GIST cases that have very complex mechanisms of drug resistance, neither imatinib nor sunitinib may be able to treat all of the highly mutated forms of KIT within aggressively behaving tumors. These would require yet another drug (a triangular-peg). Currently, only imatinib and sunitinib are yet approved for GISTs. In the future, as we understand more about GISTs, patients may be prescribed combinations of two or more targeted therapy drugs that can simultaneously block a wider range of defects within tumors.

Sunitinib is a member of the drugs known as **multikinase inhibitors**. Multikinase inhibitors hit a broader range of protein targets, and this allows these drugs to shut off more of the processes driving the cancer to grow. Besides targeting mutant KIT protein in GIST cells, sunitinib also blocks a protein called VEGF receptor. This particular protein is on the surface of the noncancerous cells that form the blood vessels that feed the tumor. By blocking the VEGF receptor, sunitinib stops the formation of new blood vessels within the tumor. If the tumor does not have a sufficient supply of blood, then it cannot grow larger. Thus, sunitinib inhibits the GIST cells by stopping their mutated forms of KIT protein and the noncancerous cells in the blood vessels that feed GIST by stopping their normal VEGF receptors.

Scientists now realize that GISTs may become resistant to a single targeted therapy in numerous ways. Treatments having

Multikinase inhibitors

Drugs that block multiple kinases (proteins) within a cell.

Sunitinib inhibits the GIST cells by stopping their mutated forms of KIT protein and the noncancerous cells in the blood vessels that feed GIST by stopping their normal VEGF receptors.

a broader range of action will probably be more effective against resistant disease than precise "smart-bullet" drugs that hone into a single trait of the disease. Researchers now believe that using combinations of targeted cancer therapies (called "cocktails") or multikinase inhibitors may be the wave of the future, as these approaches can simultaneously address several abnormalities in the cancer.

Researchers now believe that using combinations of targeted cancer therapies (called "cocktails") or multikinase inhibitors may be the wave of the future.

81. Should I discontinue the current targeted therapy if my tumor has grown? Will all of my tumors become resistant at once?

If your tumor is progressing, continued therapy might still be better than no treatment at all. Abruptly stopping all forms of targeted therapy when drug resistance becomes apparent might be a bad choice if there are no special complications or circumstances that require this. A cancer's resistance to a specific drug is not generally an all-or-nothing situation. At times, a limited subset of tumors acquires resistance to a drug, whereas the rest of your tumors continue to be held in check.

If your tumor is progressing, continued therapy might still be better than no treatment at all.

Because cancer cells are genetically unstable, over time, a few GIST cells in your body can gain additional abnormalities independently from the other GIST cells. This can cause one tumor to become resistant while your drug still controls others. Stopping therapy entirely without using an alternative therapy allows all of the GIST cells in your body to grow aggressively. In this case, what might have been a partial drug resistance and limited disease progression can become widespread progression.

You and your oncologist should take measures immediately to deal with disease progression—either through treatment modification or a different targeted therapy. Tumors with drug resistance can grow aggressively and be life threatening. Your goal is to restore complete control over your disease.

82. What should I do if the tumors are resistant to my targeted therapy?

This depends on the growth pattern in which disease progression occurs after drug resistance develops. Sometimes only one or a few tumors are progressing, but others are still responding. In other cases, widespread growth in numerous tumors is present.

Patients who have progressed on the standard 400 mg/day dose of imatinib should consider an increase to 600 or 800 mg daily before switching to another drug such as sunitinib. About a third of patients progressing at the 400 mg dose restore control over their disease by increasing their imatinib dose to 800 mg. The benefits are mostly disease stabilization, although some tumors even shrink. Patients with exon 9 *KIT* mutations are most likely to benefit from an increase in imatinib. For some reason, GISTs that are driven by exon 9 *KIT* mutations seem to respond less well to a 400 mg dose of imatinib than other GISTs with exon 11 *KIT* mutations.

If a high dose of imatinib has failed, a patient should consider switching to sunitinib. Patients with exon 9 *KIT* mutations are more likely to benefit from sunitinib after developing resistance to imatinib than those patients with exon 11 *KIT* mutations; however, many patients with exon 11 *KIT* mutations also regain disease control from sunitinib after imatinib resistance.

Currently, the only targeted cancer therapies that are available through a doctor's prescription are imatinib and sunitinib. Patients who have disease resistant to both of these drugs should consider enrolling in clinical trials of new experimental targeted cancer therapies (see Questions 85–88). Clinical trials are currently investigating agents that block the KIT protein (or alternatively PDGFRA) and their downstream signaling pathways or else drugs that prevent the growth of blood vessels.

When progression is restricted to just one or a few tumors, then surgery may be indicated. Sometimes continuation of the same drug after surgery at an increased dose can be helpful (provided that a higher dose is feasible and safe). RFA and embolization can sometimes be effective against limited sites of progression in the liver. Surgical removal or localized destruction of resistant tumors may prolong survival in patients with metastatic disease provided that the remaining disease continues to respond to drugs.

Patients who have developed widespread resistant tumors will usually not benefit much from surgery, as removing all traces of the progressing disease will be difficult. Because any tumor cells not removed during surgery will grow back quickly without effective drug treatment, these patients often have to start a new drug regimen as soon as possible.

83. What are some statistics about drug resistance?

Researchers gather statistics about the use of drugs in patients through scientifically designed clinical trials. A phase II clinical trial in 2000 was the first to test imatinib against inoperable GISTs for 147 patients. Six years later, this trial and subsequent larger phase III trials continue to track the participating patients. Certain patients have managed to go 6 years without any signs of imatinib resistance, although most patients by this time have encountered resistance.

Data from clinical trials show that

- Approximately 15% of patients have primary resistance to imatinib, meaning that their disease did not benefit at the beginning of therapy. The remaining 85% received benefit from the drug.
- At 2 years, half of all patients who started imatinib (including those with primary resistance) have experienced some form of tumor growth.

Surgical removal or localized destruction of resistant tumors may prolong survival in patients with metastatic disease provided that the remaining disease continues to respond to drugs.

Researchers gather statistics about the use of drugs in patients through scientifically designed clinical trials.

- At 2 years, about three fourths of all patients who started imatinib continued to survive, which includes the statistics for those 15% of patients who had no initial benefits. Patients with primary resistance had worse overall survival odds. For those 85% of patients who did receive a long-term benefit from imatinib, about two thirds of them continued to survive at 4 years. Overall survival statistics from a clinical trial also incorporate the survival of patients who have moved on to other therapies. As doctors have more options in the future to treat imatinib-resistant GISTs, the overall survival statistics for patients will likely improve further.

A large phase III trial conducted largely during 2004 showed that sunitinib significantly extended the time of disease control for imatinib-resistant patients compared with no therapy at all.

- Overall, two thirds of the patients who try sunitinib after becoming resistant to imatinib receive some additional disease control, mostly stability.
- Half of all of the imatinib-resistant patients trying sunitinib continued to be stable at 27 weeks. In contrast, half of the patients having no therapy suffered measurable tumor growth by 6 weeks.
- Half of the imatinib-resistant patients taking sunitinib survived to 19 months.
- At this time, no comprehensive data are available to show how well sunitinib might work in GISTs as the first treatment instead of as follow-up therapy after imatinib has failed. Sunitinib had favorable results in a few patients who were intolerant of imatinib rather than resistant to it.

These quoted statistics are overall for all cases of GISTs. Although it is not yet possible to predict accurately how any one individual patient will fare on a therapy, researchers have discovered that the clinical benefits of imatinib or sunitinib in resistant disease tend to correlate to the type of mutation (or lack of a mutation) in the *KIT* or *PDGFRA* genes. GISTs having a primary mutation in exon 11 of the *KIT* gene generally have the most favorable benefits from imatinib. Conversely, patients having a primary mutation in exon 9 of the *KIT* gene or no mutation have better responses to sunitinib in situations in which imatinib is not working.

84. Will a mutational analysis of my relapsed tumors provide useful information for selecting a new treatment?

So far, the testing for genetic mutations in GIST has remained largely a research tool for investigational clinical trials.

To give the short answer: maybe. So far, the testing for genetic mutations in GIST has remained largely a research tool for investigational clinical trials. We now know that the outcome to imatinib or sunitinib correlates somewhat to the location of the primary mutation within the tumor's *KIT* and *PDGFRA* genes. While mutational analysis of your primary tumor can help you and your doctor estimate your potential drug response, the analysis of resistance causing mutations in a relapsed tumor is mainly useful as a tool for the researcher. As the cancer becomes drug resistant, the situation on the genetic level becomes much more complicated. This is particularly true because different tumors in the same patient can develop completely different "secondary" mutations in addition to whatever mutation was present in the tumor to start. Also, because of the experimental nature of clinical trials, and certain Federal rules set up to ensure patient safety, the mutational data generated by most clinical research trials are not generally available to the patient or treating physician, and these mutational data should not be used to make any treatment decisions. Unless a clinical laboratory is performing the mutational testing under strictly controlled conditions, known as "CLIA certified conditions," the results should never be used for patient care. The U.S. Congress passed the Clinical Laboratory Improvement Amendments (CLIA) in 1988 establishing quality standards for all laboratory testing to ensure the accuracy, reliability, and timeliness of patient test results.

Many patients are interested in having mutational analysis of the *KIT* and *PDGFA* genes for their own information and peace of mind. There are a handful of laboratories worldwide which offer CLIA-certified mutational analysis of GIST, pioneered by Drs. Christopher Corless and Michael Heinrich in the pathology department of the Oregon Health and Sciences University, Portland, Oregon. It is possible that in the future this information might be useful when making difficult clinical decisions, such as the optimal selection of targeted therapy or whether surgery should be performed. We can expect the usefulness of clinical diagnostic mutational analysis to increase in the future as more is understood about resistant GISTs and there are more proven treatments for them. It is likely that we will eventually see the mutational status of a patient's tumors as a crucial tool to match a patient to the drug (or drugs) that has the greatest efficacy for the specific mutation involved. However, that time has not yet arrived. But for now, overall, the treatment options for GIST patients are limited, and so we are not yet ready for personalized cancer therapy based on detailed mutational information.

85. What is a clinical trial, and who is eligible to participate?

A clinical trial is a research study that allows physicians to answer specific medical questions. Medical researchers discover new therapies daily and describe their mode of action with an evolving precision. To establish safety and efficacy, those newly discovered therapies must be tested in patients.

Clinical trials test new drugs, a combination of known drugs, the method of administering certain drugs, and new therapies. All clinical trials are and should always be detailed and clearly described in a **protocol**, which describes all of the rules and conditions that govern the trial. This ensures the quality of the trial and thus its reproducibility, as well as the safety and protection of the patients on the trial.

Protocol

The ultimate reference for clinical trials that describes all the rules and conditions that govern the trial; ensures the quality of the trial and thus its reproducibility, as well as the safety and protection of the patients in the trial.

Unfortunately, history tells us about badly conducted clinical trials that might have exploited patients for the sake of answering a scientific question. Nowadays, patients should not fear joining a clinical trial when clinically indicated, as federal regulations that protect all patients now govern all protocols. An institutional review board monitors these rules and many other ethical considerations very closely. Patients who are given an opportunity to join a clinical trial ultimately choose whether to participate. If the patient enters a trial, he or she has the right to withdraw at any time. The patient and physician should discuss these rights and the details of the study in a process called **informed consent**, which culminates in the signing of an agreement. This ensures the coherence of the study and protects the rights of all patients.

Clinical trials generally happen in three phases: **phase I, phase II**, and **phase III**. A phase I study primarily establishes the safety of a newly discovered drug or a combination of drugs, while studying the efficacy in many diseases. Phase II trials primarily study the efficacy of a drug or a combination of drugs in a specific disease; however, the ultimate answer on efficacy is usually sought through a phase III study, which compares the experimental drug or drugs to the standard care of this disease. In a phase III trial, patients are randomly assigned to experimental versus standard care to ensure the validity of the experiment.

86. Where can I find about clinical trials for GIST, and how do I know which trial is best for me?

Ask your doctors about clinical trials. Many doctors at academic centers and in private offices participate in clinical trials. Patients might consider commuting a reasonable distance to get to a center that runs a pertinent clinical trial. Patients can learn about those either through their doctors, the center website, or through the government National Cancer Institute (NCI) websites (www.cancer.gov and www.clinicaltrials.gov). The NCI offers not only a listing of all clinical trials that are

Informed consent

When a patient agrees to a certain procedure or treatment by signing an agreement that says the patient understands the procedure or treatment, the risks, and benefits and that the rights and safety of the patient have been discussed.

Phase I

The study that primarily establishes the safety of a newly discovered drug or a combination of drugs, while studying the efficacy in many diseases.

Phase II

The study that primarily evaluates the efficacy of a drug or a combination of drugs in a specific disease.

Phase III

The study that compares the experimental drug or drugs with the standard care of this disease or a placebo.

registered with them, but also several websites with information about clinical trials. Other sites that offer similar services include the Coalition of National Cancer Cooperative Groups (www.cancertrialshelp.org) and Centerwatch (www.centerwatch.com).

If a patient identifies a relevant clinical trial, he or she should discuss the trial further with his or her doctor. The doctor can call the investigators and find out more about the trial. This ensures that patients participate in only trials for which they are eligible and thus save a lot of frustration, travel time, and expenses. If a patient is deemed ineligible for a certain trial, he or she should not be disappointed or feel hopeless. Certain clinical trials answer only a specific question in a specific subset of patients with a given disease.

Ask your doctors about clinical trials. Many doctors at academic centers and in private offices participate in clinical trials.

87. What are the potential risks and benefits from participating in a clinical trial?

Like most treatments in the current health care environment, risks and benefits exist when participating in a clinical trial. Although clinical trials may give you access to the latest proposed treatments and the benefit of an effective therapy for your cancer, clinical trials can also have additional risks.

Almost all treatments carry risk, and unproven treatments in clinical trials for patients with GIST are no different. The therapies or combination of therapies will carry the risk of side effects and adverse reactions. Some of these side effects and adverse reactions are expected, but some can be unexpected. You can even die from some of the reactions. You could also be assigned to the placebo group, which means that you would not be exposed to risk, but you would also not receive any of the benefits from the new treatment.

The obvious benefit of participating in a clinical trial is that a treatment might improve your condition. This benefit has to be weighed with the risks, especially that you could become sicker.

Not all of the benefits pertain directly to you. Clinical trials provide you with the chance to do something that could eventually benefit many people. Some people who decide to participate in clinical trials believe that doing so gives them greater control over their health care. Sometimes participation in a trial gives you more frequent contact with a team of people who care for you as well.

By weighing the benefits and risks of a clinical trial, you will be making an informed decision. After you are enrolled in a clinical trial, you have the right to withdraw or decline further participation.

88. What are the expenses for participating in a clinical trial?

Some trials will cover travel expenses and the additional physician visits that are needed to evaluate your response. Most drugs and treatments that are being researched are provided at no cost. Most insurance plans cover the appointments and tests that you normally would have had if you had not participated in the trial. Always ask about expenses when you are interviewed for the trial. Also, be sure to check with your insurance carrier before you agree to participate. Many private insurers, although sometimes reluctant to pay for clinical trials, will examine the merits of each case individually. Medicare will cover the routine expenses associated with phase II and phase III government-sponsored clinical trials.

Because private health insurance carriers have previously perceived clinical trials as too experimental and therefore too risky, many states have now passed laws pertaining to clinical trials. The American Cancer Society has up-to-date information about legislative action at the state and federal level (www.cancer.org/docroot/ETO/content/ETO_6_2x_State_Laws_Regarding_Clinical_Trials.asp). Question 100 provides resources for additional information about clinical trials.

PART ELEVEN

Social and End-of-Life Issues

My disease is progressing. How do I decide when it is time to stop looking for other types of treatments? What is the best supportive care?

Should targeted cancer therapy continue even though the disease has become terminal?

How can I become free of pain? Will I become addicted to pain medications?

More . . .

89. My disease is progressing. How do I decide when it is time to stop looking for other types of treatments? What is the best supportive care?

If your cancer becomes too advanced and resistant to therapy or if your body becomes too weak to tolerate further treatment, your doctor may decide to minimize your therapies and provide supportive care instead. This does not mean that your doctor has given up and is withdrawing treatment. The best supportive care means that your doctor focuses on reducing your symptoms. You will still see your doctor regularly and discuss pain control, nutrition, and other symptoms or concerns.

Families may not easily recognize that further aggressive treatments should be stopped. Because one patient's cancer affects the entire family unit, some members may be slower to accept the decision and even accuse other family members of giving up hope too soon. This can compound an already tense situation. In some circumstances, family members should even encourage a weary patient to keep trying. Nevertheless, the family must try to accept the patient's decision. Despite family conflict, the decision to stop aggressive therapy is deeply personal. The disease itself will take charge of the situation regardless.

For enduring peace of mind, crucial decisions must be made with full awareness of the most up-to-date information about clinical trials possibilities, of the most recent clinical practice guidelines for GISTs, and with the best medical advice.

90. Should targeted cancer therapy continue even though the disease has become terminal?

You should not necessarily quit taking targeted cancer therapy entirely, even if you have accepted that your disease is **terminal** and you are prepared to receive end-of-life support

If your cancer becomes too advanced and resistant to therapy or if your body becomes too weak to tolerate further treatment, your doctor may decide to minimize your therapies and provide supportive care instead.

Terminal

Disease that cannot be cured and will cause death.

care. Drugs that inhibit the KIT protein, such as imatinib or sunitinib, may slow the growth of some tumors even while the disease overall progresses.

The reason for this is rooted in the complex nature of GIST. All of the individual GIST cells within your entire tumor load are not entirely genetically identical. Cancer cells are notoriously negligent at repairing any damage that occurs in their DNA. Your tumor began with a single cancerous cell, but numerous subsequent rounds of cell division created masses of cells that may have genetically wandered away from each other over time. Your targeted therapy may continue to control some subpopulations of GIST cells even as drug-resistant subpopulations have emerged, causing overall growth of particular tumors. Completely quitting your targeted therapy altogether may allow all of the GIST cells in your body to divide, thus making the disease worse. Moreover, sometimes trying the targeted cancer therapy that you took previously but stopped taking in order to try another drug may bring an additional measure of disease control.

Your targeted therapy may continue to control some subpopulations of GIST cells even as drug-resistant subpopulations have emerged, causing overall growth of particular tumors. Completely quitting your targeted therapy altogether may allow all of the GIST cells in your body to divide, thus making the disease worse.

Continuing cancer therapy even though the tumors progress is not the way that oncologists typically manage patients who are taking traditional chemotherapies. Some terminally ill GIST patients should stay on targeted cancer therapy because of the relatively mild side effects and because some of the GIST cells may continue to be controlled, although the overall disease progression is not stopped. Discuss with your oncologist whether the benefits of taking the drug outweigh the side effects.

91. How can I become free of pain? Will I become addicted to pain medications?

Pain must be controlled so that it doesn't affect your mood, function, and energy level. Numerous pain-management medications are available. Mild pain usually responds to acetaminophen (Tylenol) or nonsteroidal anti-inflammatory

Pain must be controlled so that it doesn't affect your mood, function, and energy level.

drugs such as Motrin or Advil. Use Tylenol sparingly, as it may harm your liver if you are also taking a tyrosine kinase inhibitor. The major risk of nonsteroidal anti-inflammatory drugs is stomach inflammation or bleeding.

Narcotic-based medications, which come in short- and long-acting forms, are required for more severe pain. Oxycodone is a short-acting agent, and generally, you can take one to two pills every 4 to 6 hours. Oxycodone is also combined with Tylenol in a medication called Percocet. Your doctor may want to limit the use of Percocet because it contains Tylenol. If you have a lot of pain, long-acting opiates include Oxycontin or MS Contin, which are taken twice a day. Alternatively, Fentanyl, a skin patch, can be applied every 3 days.

The common side effects of opiates include fatigue and constipation. A stool softener like Colace or a laxative like Senekot or Magnesium citrate or Lactulose will most likely be needed. Do not drive while taking opiates. Some experimenting may be necessary to determine which formulation and dose best control your pain and minimize your side effects. Your requirement for pain medications may increase because you may develop tolerance. Tolerance is natural and is distinct from addiction. Addiction is a set of behaviors that focuses on constantly seeking the drug.

92. What is Hospice?

Hospice is a philosophy about end-of-life care—not a specific place of care. Hospice is appropriate when a patient can no longer benefit from cancer treatments and has a limited life expectancy, generally 6 months or less. Hospice helps to maintain the quality of life during the last stages of an incurable disease.

Hospice care focuses on the management of pain and other symptoms. It also attends to the spiritual, emotional, and social needs of dying patients and their families. Most hospice

Narcotic

A potent drug derived from opium or opium-like compounds given to relieve pain; associated with significant effects on mood and behavior with the potential for dependence and tolerance.

Hospice

A philosophy about end-of-life care, not a specific place of care; appropriate when a patient can no longer benefit from cancer treatments and has a limited life expectancy, generally 6 months or less. The principal aim is to maintain quality of life during the last stages of incurable disease.

Hospice helps to maintain the quality of life during the last stages of an incurable disease.

services in the United States are based in the patient's home, where a family member provides round-the-clock supervision and much of the hands-on care. Hospice care is also offered in inpatient hospice centers, nursing homes, and hospitals.

Hospice care uses an interdisciplinary health care team of physicians, nurses, social workers, counselors, home health aides, clergy, therapists, and trained volunteers. The interdisciplinary team coordinates and supervises all aspects of care. The hospice nurse and sometimes a hospice physician make regularly scheduled visits to check on the patient's condition, provide pain management, and arrange for needed medical equipment. Social workers and other team members offer assistance with practical and financial concerns, emotional counseling for the entire family, and bereavement follow-up. Sometimes a health aide is needed in the home to help with daily activities such as bathing and eating.

When it is time to start thinking about hospice arrangements? After a cancer diagnosis, you might want to gather in advance the necessary information about the hospice programs that are available in your area. Your physician or hospital social worker can help with this. Also, contact your state's departments of health or social services to obtain a list of licensed agencies, or contact the state hospice organization. The state health department oversees certification of hospice services.

Admission to hospice generally requires a hospice team member to visit the home to learn about your situation. By law, the decision to join a hospice belongs to the patient, who will be asked to sign consent forms. The decision to sign up for hospice may come with confusing feelings and expectations. Accepting hospice care does not mean that you are giving up hope or that your death will be hastened. Instead, remember that under hospice care, a patient receives specialized assistance to cope with end-stage disease, and family members can receive appropriate services as well. Furthermore, a patient may be able to receive certain cancer therapies to alleviate symptoms and remain eligible for hospice. Patients who show signs of improvement may elect to leave hospice and return to more aggressive therapy.

Health insurance plans pay some hospice expenses, and medical costs that insurance does not cover are sometimes tax deductible. Check with your health insurance provider about coverage. Medicare insurance provides coverage for hospice care, and a list of Medicare-certified hospice programs is available through your state health department. See the list of resources for hospice in Question 100.

93. How much time do I have left? Should I ask my doctor to make this prediction?

This is one of the first questions that patients ask when they are diagnosed with cancer. Studies have examined the accuracies of these life expectancy predictions. Results showed that doctors have difficulty predicting exact times, but they do have a sense of when things are going wrong. The nearer a patient is to death, the more accurate is the prediction. One study found that long-term clinical estimates beyond 6 months had no predictive value. In short-term situations, the clinical predictions were correct to within a week 25% of the time and correct to within 4 weeks in 61% of cases. Doctors most frequently overestimated survival. Nevertheless, their overestimations tended to correlate in a proportional manner to the actual survival outcome.

Rather than asking him precisely how long you have to live, depersonalize the implications by asking your doctor for relevant statistics about your particular situation.

Your prognosis is the fundamental basis for how you react to your cancer situation. It defines whether to accept aggressive treatments or comfort care. It shapes your emotional state and how you plan your affairs. A balance exists between the benefits of knowing versus not knowing the doctor's prediction of your life expectancy. An accurate prediction can rally appropriate responses. An inaccurate estimate may pull you into regrettable decisions or lead to emotional fluctuations. Some patients just do not want to know or would cope better without knowing. Their thoughts may overwhelm their ability to focus on the remaining days.

As a patient, you need to know the seriousness of your situation so that you can respond suitably. Rather than asking him precisely how long you have to live, depersonalize the implications by asking your doctor for relevant statistics about your particular situation. Base your decisions about care on these statistics, while centering your emotional state on Dr. Stephen Jay Gould's hopeful essay "The Median is not the Message," which can be found at cancerguide.org/median_not_msg. html.

94. What are advance health care directives?

Patients have the right to control their medical treatment and even refuse treatment. **Advance health care directives**, more commonly called advance directives, refer to your oral and written instructions about your medical care if you become unable to communicate. To protect your wishes before you become seriously ill, prepare legal written instructions that document what you want for future medical care. Designate a person to act in your behalf. You do not need a lawyer to prepare advance directives. Check with your local hospital or health department for the appropriate forms. Once drafted, the advance directives should be signed, dated, witnessed, notarized, and incorporated into your medical record. Also, arrange for these advance directives to be distributed to your authorized surrogate, family, and friends.

Two basic types of advance directives exist: a **health care proxy** and a **living will**. A health care proxy is a person appointed to make the medical decisions if the patient is unable to do so. As long as the patient is still able to communicate his or her wishes, he or she always retains the authority to

Advance health care directives

Your oral and written instructions about your medical care in the event you become unable to communicate for yourself; includes a health care proxy and a living will.

Two basic types of advance directives exist: a health care proxy and a living will.

Health care proxy

A person appointed to make a patient's medical decisions if the patient is unable to do so.

Living will

Specific instructions regarding measures that would prolong life, outlining the medical interventions to be performed or withheld, including life-sustaining procedures or artificial life support in the event the patient can no longer communicate.

make the decisions. Ask someone to be your proxy. Be sure to choose someone you trust and someone who will follow your preferences—not his or her own. A health care proxy may have to exercise his or her own judgment if the patient's wishes are not known for a particular medical procedure. Communicate in detail with your proxy about what you would want in a variety of circumstances, and confirm that he or she is willing to honor these wishes. It is also a good idea to name an alternate person. The **durable power of attorney for health care** is the only legal document that authorizes a person to serve as a patient's health care proxy. An ordinary power of attorney gives another person the legal right to conduct business matters in your name for you, but does not give another person the legal right to make decisions about your medical care.

Durable power of attorney for health care

The legal document that authorizes a person to serve as a patient's health care proxy.

A living will outlines your choices for health care if you become terminally ill or permanently unconscious. A living will is more limited than a durable power of attorney for health care. A living will applies only when there is no hope for recovery. In a living will, you can state specific instructions about measures that would prolong your life, outlining the medical interventions you would want performed or have withheld. This removes the burden of making these decisions from family, friends and physicians. Types of life-sustaining care include the use of equipment, such as dialysis machines, ventilators, and respirators, and the administration of blood products, certain medications, artificial hydration, and nutrition.

Cardiopulmonary resuscitation

A series of actions and treatments that are used when a patient is no longer breathing or no longer has a pulse.

In the advanced stages of cancer, your heart and lungs may stop. Unless given other instructions, hospital staff and emergency medical teams will try to help those patients. Specify in advance whether you want **cardiopulmonary resuscitation**, electric shock to your heart, special medications to restart your heart, and the insertion of a plastic tube in your throat to allow you to be connected to a ventilator. In the case of advanced cancer, these heroic interventions are likely to fail. If anything, they may be tormenting, painful, and nondignifying to you and your family. In those instances, your doctor may recommend that you approve a **Do-Not-Resuscitate (DNR), Do-Not-Intubate (DNI) order**. Of course, the decision is yours and is an important part of your advance directives. Have an open and frank discussion with your doctor about DNR/DNI orders to make sure that you understand them. Also, make sure that you have informed your health care proxy of your decision. A DNR/DNI order does not limit your access to medical care and is different from hospice care.

Regulations on advance directives vary by state. The decisions of health care proxies and living wills may not be recognized in all states. Before preparing your advance directives, check with your state's health department. Some people believe that after the advance directives have been signed, they cannot be changed. In fact, your advance directives can be modified or withdrawn at any time.

Mary's (closest family member of a patient without advance directives) comments:

Suppose that you have a loved one in the hospital who is very ill and who has never been married or had any children—only siblings. This person is incoherent and unconscious most of the time. You, as the closest family member, want to help and care for this person. You ask the doctor what the prognosis is, what treatment is being given, and what are the chances for recovery. The doctor cannot answer your questions, stating that the privacy laws do not allow him to reveal this information without the patient's written permission signed before a witness. The hospital staff says the same thing. The loved ones who are wanting to help feel very frustrated over and over again. If the patient had created a power of attorney for heath care, appointing a trusted loved one to make decisions and gather information, the relationship between the family and medical providers would be more positive.

Social and End-of-Life Issues

Do-Not-Resuscitate (DNR) order

An advance directive that says that CPR should not be performed in the event the patient stops breathing or no longer has a pulse.

Do-Not-Intubate (DNI) order

An advance directive that says that the patient should not be intubated (with a plastic mouthpiece and tube) in the event that the patient stops breathing or no longer has a pulse.

95. What is anticipatory grief?

Dr. Therese Rando, PhD, has written extensively about the psychology of loss and grief. She observes, "Anticipatory grief is not merely conventional post-death grief begun earlier." Instead, anticipatory grief covers the complicated set of emotional reactions and practical adaptations by a family during the lengthy period leading up to the loss of a loved one. Dealing with a prolonged terminal illness calls for a delicate balance among conflicting demands, "drawing close to the dying loved one and simultaneously letting go of him or her." Anticipatory grief affects all aspects of a family: emotional, social, interpersonal, spiritual, financial, physical, and developmental states. Family members face major changes in their lives and try to find some way of coming to terms. Feelings similar to post-death grieving are also part of the experience.

A "good" anticipatory grief can be therapeutic, as family members gradually absorb the reality of the imminent death and complete unfinished business with the dying person; however, too much grieving can have negative effects, such as social withdrawal, poor communications, and premature emotional separations between the family and dying person. Not all families feel anticipatory grief, and this is also normal. Not everyone in a family will go through the last days of cancer with the same reactions. Counseling services, religious organizations, or people in your community can lend a hand to your family.

Dr. Betty Davies, RN, PhD, is a leading researcher in the fields of dying, death, and bereavement. She describes two distinct perspectives of anticipatory grief: that of the dying individual and that of all others who care about him or her. A patient grapples with becoming increasingly dependent on others as his or her physical capabilities diminish. Patients often describe the final days as a surreal "fading away." A dying person wrestles with letting go of everyone he or she has known, and he or she may feel disconnected from the world.

Anticipatory grief

Covers the complicated set of emotional reactions and practical adaptations by a family during the lengthy period leading up to the loss of a loved one.

Dealing with a prolonged terminal illness calls for a delicate balance among conflicting demands, "drawing close to the dying loved one and simultaneously letting go of him or her."

The family is called on to handle extra responsibilities and to prepare for a future without the loved one. Caregivers can become drained from the stresses of caring for a dying loved one. They may feel emotionally numb at the time of death or harbor guilty feelings because they doubt their love for the deceased. When a patient is able to acknowledge that he or she is dying and adjust the outlook accordingly, then his or her family can to deal with the situation more effectively. If a family member remains unwilling to accept what is happening, then tensions arise, as the family cannot address the effects of the illness.

A prolonged state of sadness can overwhelm a dying person's self-perception about his or her identity or can seem to erase the connection to his or her past life. Strive to recognize the happy memories, and avoid assigning blame for the past. Mend fences if possible. Sometimes a dying person finds solace in mapping out plans for his or her family's future. These thoughts can be comforting for a dying person who is dress rehearsing for the future and indirectly placing himself or herself in it. The age and developmental states of children determine how anticipatory grief affects them. Younger children do not readily grasp the permanency of death, and their anxiety levels are likely determined from their own parents' reactions. Teenagers may lack some of the abilities to look into the future, and hence may pass up the opportunity to draw closer to their dying parent.

How a family reacts in the days leading up to the death of their loved one is determined mostly by their circumstances before the illness. Factors such as socioeconomics, culture, religious beliefs, interpersonal dynamics, and individual psychology all come into the picture. Sometimes a terminal prognosis may deepen pre-existing problems in the family. Our attitudes about dying are shaped not so much by our age but whether we believe that we have accomplished most of our life's goals or if we are leaving important work unfinished. They are also shaped by our relationships to the ones we are

How a family reacts in the days leading up to the death of their loved one is determined mostly by their circumstances before the illness.

leaving behind. No single coping strategy fits every person's situation. The three most valuable reminders for these times are probably empathy, patience, and forgiveness.

Following are the voices of three individuals who each bring a different perspective about coping during a terminal illness: the spouse, the elementary school–aged son, and the mother dying from metastatic GIST. The family history is unusual because the GIST patient eventually recovered fully after having been close to death. Several years later, Keith describes his role as a caregiver, giving practical advice on how to maintain family balance. Kevin, once the young son, now describes his quest to have a normal childhood in the face of the chaos that the cancer brought. Marina, the dying patient, feels disconnected from the world.

Keith's (spouse of a hospice patient) comments:

There are no pat answers to this question, as everyone is different. Aristotle's maxim that moderation in all things is best is probably the best answer. You do the sick person no good if you become so prostrate with grief that you cannot function, but you equally do them no good if you deny them their experience with illness. People react differently as the cancer progresses. Remember that the anger, the tears, the grief are not directed at you, even though it may seem like you are the target.

Just as the patient needs someone to help him work through these issues, so will you when the time comes. You will know how you deal with grief, and it may not be the way your loved one does. Try to avoid these types of grief conflicts with the patient. Find another friend or relative to talk it through with, or get a counselor to work you through these issues. Although they don't advertise it, many health insurance companies will pay for counseling to help you and any minor children.

As your loved gets closer to death, more of your time and energy may be spent caring for the sick person. You must find time for yourself, as you must have the space to deal with your own grief issues. The patient will also feel this constriction of his or her world, as he or she becomes weaker and less able to interact socially. This often leads to the patient becoming more emotionally needy and leaning on you, the caregiver. A balance exists that you must find on your own between the needs of the patient, the needs of the rest of your immediate family (if you have small children), and your own needs. People will try to tell you where that balance point should be, but you are the only one who can really know your own emotional boundaries. Find someone who is a good listener, and talk these issues out until you find the line with which you are comfortable.

Kevin's (young son of a hospice patient) comments:

When I was 10 years old my mother was diagnosed with advanced terminal GIST. I never had difficulty accepting that my mother was sick, although as a youth, the prospect of death was so alien as to seem impossible. The emotional turbulence in my house shaped my perceptions about my mother much more than the cancer itself. You do your child or loved ones no favors by giving into despair or anger.

Eventually my mother was enrolled in hospice when I was 12. Still, I had to develop as a normal middle-school kid with typical school experiences. Our father had to work, and thus, my siblings and I were left on our own for much of the time while our mother was bedridden. As the eldest, I took up much of the burden of caring for my brother and sister who were very young. I learned to build relationships with members of our community who were willing to act as a surrogate family during this time of crisis. I sometimes feel as though my childhood rearing was as much a product of my community as of my parents. Through prolonged adversity, I gained a self-reliance that has benefited me ever since.

One of the best ways of handling the grief of approaching loss is to get involved. Join your local church (or mosque or synagogue) youth group. Sign up for school activities, and volunteer your time

*to your community. It's truly amazing how many caring and lov-
ing people there are in the world if only you spend the energy to
meet them. My community became my surrogate family when and
wherever my immediate family could not be, and that relationship
has blossomed into one of the most important in my life as I now
enter adulthood.*

Marina's (hospice patient, wife of Keith, and mother of Kevin)
comments:

*I was diagnosed with metastastic GIST before effective drug treat-
ments were available. I endured 3 years without any hope, 8
months in hospice, and a very near brush with death. I would
eventually recover after imatinib became available in year 2000,
and years of good health have since followed. I do not feel any
lasting stress about my time in hospice, but rather, I am left with
optimism about the resilience of the human spirit. Nevertheless,
I do have recollections about what it is like to be a dying person
during prolonged illness.*

*There is something incomprehensible about your own death, even
as you intellectually know that it is imminent. If you feel as though
you are "dying before your time," then you can never entirely resolve
your utter disbelief. Lacking any internal resolution, there became
two versions of me within one body. First was my inner-voice
companion who was the person I had always been. I co-existed
with a stranger who was an invalid cancer patient, both of us
trapped in a sinking vessel. During the hospice days, I said many
times, "I do not want to watch what is happening to me," as though
I was an observer from the sidelines.*

*Everyone appreciates how a terminal illness cuts a person off
from the future; however, I did not anticipate was how much the
diagnosis would cut me off from my past. So much of my past was
inextricably intertwined with assumptions about a future now
entirely derailed by the cancer. My perceptions about my past life
became curiously distorted by a filter of sadness. In this regard, I
felt cut off from both my past and my future.*

The only way for friends or family to connect with me was to make a connection into my cancer and to share my despair. This would require them to leave their own reality of good health for a while to experience dying in a vicarious way. Demanding an intense witnessing of tragedy for months on end is a lot to ask of someone who is otherwise leading a comfortable life. At many points, exhausted supporters would ask that I just try to embrace the life that I did have, as it was dealt to me, so that they might have a little break from my ordeal.

Having been healthy once and then abruptly terminally ill, I came to realize that there are divergent perspectives about life's routines and its celebrations. Probably no heart is more broken than that of a terminally ill cancer patient with young children who has been called on to stand next to a Christmas tree and pose for pictures. Pointing out our inability to cooperate in good spirits will compound our sense of failure. I see no easy away around the needs of the dying to shield themselves from observances that remind them of what will be lost versus the needs of the healthy to have memories and photos. Ideally, the more you can do to build good memories for the children is better. But nothing about hospice rates as "ideally." Playing a card game with your young children while in your bed and taking photographs at the time can be easier for you. It celebrates the moment within the scope of the hospice patient, which usually is limited to the confines of his bedroom. Asking a dying person, "Don't you want to get dressed and go outside?" is sometimes asking too much from the patient.

Making what you can out of the days in hospice requires focusing only in the present—and that may mean not looking past the hour before you. If the day mandates making your bedroom the entirety of the universe, then so be it. A hospice patient must downsize the scale of his world so that everything about it does not seem so beyond his reach. Emotional pain comes if your ever-constricting circumstances are laid bare against wide-open images of healthy vigor and the future. To the caregivers, don't expect your dying loved one to behave as though he or she is integrated in a world that tends to be ordered around the perspectives of the healthy. Respect that your loved one is busy "fading away," and he or she needs to do that by gradually exiting your life via stage left.

96. What should I do to prepare to die? What are the end stages of GIST like?

Some GIST patients have thought that they had reached the end of life and were thus using hospice care; but then, they were given a lifesaving treatment. Not everyone can expect something so dramatic. After your tumors progress and become resistant to all the known therapies, you must have a frank discussion with your physician about what to expect. You will probably want to discuss the following: how much pain you can expect and how the pain will be managed, which of your organ systems will shut down first, what kind of symptoms will you have, what happens to your breathing (and not just that you will stop breathing eventually), and how you will know that death is imminent so that you can have loved ones around you.

After your tumors progress and become resistant to all the known therapies, you must have a frank discussion with your physician about what to expect.

Death is the natural conclusion of life. Although you may fear death, preparing for it might help to make a smooth transition. Thinking of death does not mean giving up. Instead, it helps you shape how your life will end. Preparing earlier is better.

Settle your financial issues. Work with your attorney, accountant, and your family. You may need to write a will, especially if your family is financially dependent on you. Sort out your financial plan, and keep your attorney's name and contacts available. Also, make sure to keep all legal, financial, or health documents organized.

See your loved ones, family, friends, and colleagues. Talk to people who live far away. If any unresolved issues with somebody trouble you, work on settling them. Indicate to whom you want to give your valuable items. Collectibles and photographs are memories that will celebrate your life and may be passed from one generation to another. You may wish to prepare some aspects of your funeral. This is a celebration of your life and an important closure for everybody.

The biggest remaining fear is leaving your loved ones, especially children, behind. See them as often as you can. Prepare an album of photos about your life. Leave your scrapbooks or diaries, as this will be a comfort to them.

As you can imagine, you might be busy even close to your death. Remember and recite to yourself your dearest moments. You will notice that you are abundant with life.

97. What should families consider about facing bereavement?

According to J. William Worden, who has written extensively about grief, four principal tasks are essential to the mourning process: (1) accepting the reality of the loss, (2) working through the pain of grief, (3) adjusting to life without the deceased, and (4) "emotionally relocating the deceased and moving on," which does not mean forgetting the deceased, but rather finding an "appropriate place" for them "in their emotional lives—a place that will enable [those left behind] to go on living effectively in the world."

Grieving is painful. People in grief can experience feelings of sadness, anger, guilt, and/or anxiety, as well as physical sensations, such as hollowness in the stomach or tightness in the chest and tearfulness. We may have confusion, preoccupation, longing for the deceased, searching and calling out, sleep and appetite disturbances, social withdrawal, and sometimes restless hyperactivity. These reactions will normally diminish and pass with time. Talking with your family and friends, a member of the clergy, or a grief counselor can help.

In Worden's view, mourning the loss of a close relationship requires at least 1 year, but possibly 2, although this varies

People in grief can experience feelings of sadness, anger, guilt, and/or anxiety, as well as physical sensations, such as hollowness in the stomach or tightness in the chest and tearfulness.

greatly depending on the individual and cultural background. Mourning is completed when the bereaved person can think of the deceased without pain and can "reinvest his or her emotions back into life and in the living." If the grief is so intense that it leaves you feeling overwhelmed or unable to cope or if it lasts for an unusually long time, a grief specialist may help you to work toward completion of mourning. Long periods of grief can lead to clinical depression; thus, talk with a professional if you are concerned about the depth or breadth of your grief process.

As a caregiver, you may feel relief now that your caregiving responsibilities have come to an end. For some, these feelings can lead to further feelings of guilt. Others become anxious because in addition to the loss of their loved one they are losing their defining role as a caregiver. You are now embarking on your own journey of healing. Be kind to yourself, and don't forget to reach out to others to help you find your place in the world again. The authors are grateful to Susannah L. Rose, MSSW, and Richard T. Hara, PhD, authors of *100 Questions & Answers About Caring for Family or Friends with Cancer*, for this information.

PART TWELVE

The Proactive and Informed Patient

How much will self-education help me?

What should I know about patient support groups and health-related information on the Internet?

Where can I learn more information about GIST?

More . . .

98. How much will self-education help me?

Access to cancer information on the Internet has allowed us to feel more like discerning consumers of health care, and this is influencing the doctor–patient relationship. As health care consumers, we want information to guide our care. Some family members cope well by reading everything available about GIST and their treatments. Their motivation may come out of concern that they will pay greater attention to the details of their care or that no one has more to lose by oversights. Ideally, self-education about your disease can enhance your working relationship with the oncologist. You can better assimilate what he or she tells you, feel more proactive in tough decisions, and make judgments about the quality of your care.

Conversely, some patients find the extra information to be intimidating and thus compound their stress levels. They prefer the traditional doctor–patient relationship as their complete source of information. For the most part, these patients do not have a major disadvantage. A good physician, particularly one specializing in the care of GIST patients, can explain all of the important information. He or she will help you to make the best medical decisions. Although your general oncologist may not have treated many previous GIST patients, he or she can learn about the new ways of treating GIST through continuing medical education programs.

Keep informed about new clinical trials for GIST through the Internet. This can bring useful information that your oncologist may not have known about. Your general oncologist may not have the time to routinely scope out an appropriate clinical trial situation. If you find something intriguing on the Internet, then print it. Consider whether your doctor could realistically pursue this idea for you. He or she cannot act on preliminary laboratory discoveries or treatments designed for other types of cancer. Both you and your doctor should keep an open mind about the information and why it would or would not be helpful.

What you read about another GIST patient may not apply to you. GISTs and their behaviors vary among patients, and each case requires its own personalized clinical management. Also, realize that some things are simply unknowable no matter how much you have researched for more information. Medicine cannot answer how well you will respond to a particular therapy or what your future holds. Try to accept this.

If you can use at least a cartoon version to explain the simplest concepts about GIST, then you will begin to view the disease as a random biological accident and not anything that you could have brought on yourself. This awareness can release you from self-blame. You can also gain an appreciation about how your targeted therapy drug actually works.

99. What should I know about patient support groups and health-related information on the Internet?

Patient Support Groups on the Internet

Participating in an Internet patient support group or message board might be helpful for several reasons. First, GISTs are rare; thus, individuals with GIST are unlikely to meet up with each other by chance or be able to have a support group in their communities. Support groups over the Internet allow you to converse with other individuals who are in a similar situation. Second, knowledge about GIST is evolving at a rapid pace. Internet-based support groups provide approachable and informal settings where patients and their families can ask questions and learn a lot quickly. Internet groups often give their membership information about newly opened clinical trials or breaking scientific developments. Savvy members of support groups provide a wealth of useful information and insider's tips. They take on the role of mentor and teacher, distilling technical information into plain terms and helping you to hone into the most relevant information.

Internet-based support groups provide approachable and informal settings where patients and their families can ask questions and learn a lot quickly.

The benefits of peer-to-peer support can be considerable, even when the sharing arrives via cyberspace. There may be no one in your three-dimensional world who truly comprehends the challenges that a GIST diagnosis brings; perhaps no one around you is willing to take on your daily cancer-related problems. Those confronting a similar cancer diagnosis can share candid insights that come only from living with cancer. They are less likely to shy away from your cancer identity. Telling your account as you witness the stories of others is highly therapeutic. Personal illness narratives help you to redefine your expectations about the world in a way that incorporates cancer into your reality.

Keep a perspective on both the strengths and the limitations of patient support groups on the Internet. Realize that you will be corresponding with people who likely have no medical training and who are seeking community and learning just like you. Even well-intentioned people may inadvertently circulate inaccurate material or skewed opinions. Do not feel obligated to comply if someone from a patient support group requests your private medical data. Data from Internet groups are not scientific and are not useful to professionals. Privacy is never guaranteed on the Internet; thus, do not share sensitive details about yourself. See the index for a list of GIST patient organizations.

Health-Related Information on the Internet

The Pew Internet & American Life Project conducted a survey in 2005 about the Internet as a tool for handling major life events, including major medical conditions. Respondents described three roles for the Internet: (1) connecting them to other people for support and advice, (2) finding information or comparing options, and (3) finding professional or expert services. According to the survey, 24 million Americans within a 2-year period felt that the Internet had played an important role in the decision-making about major medical conditions. Only a few felt overloaded by the volume of health information.

The reliability and usefulness of the Internet's health information may range from excellent to poor, as no regulatory oversight exists. Moreover, a patient and a medical professional may have differing opinions about the helpfulness of a site. Judging whether the health content of a particular website is accurate can pose a challenge for someone who is not medically trained. No hard rules can be applied beyond your critical instincts. The National Cancer Institute (www.cancer.gov) has compiled a checklist for your consideration:

- Who sponsors the website? The sponsor pays for the cost of the website. The source of funding can affect what and how the content is presented. Take note of the ending of the web addresses: ".gov" are government sponsored, ".edu" denotes educational institutes, ".com" are commercial organizations, and ".org" indicates noncommercial organizations. Many medical centers have websites with searchable online patient education information. Nonprofit organizations can differ greatly in their operations, from established trusted names in health fields, including professional societies, to single-focus interest groups, and/or groups with small infrastructure. Look for information about who contributes to the nonprofit organization, realizing that some nonprofit organizations may have undue financial ties to special interests.
- What is the purpose of the website? Many websites have a link—"About this Site"—that is often at the bottom of the home page. This should state clearly the mission of the website and should help you to evaluate whether the site carries a particular point of view or slant.
- What type of information is presented on the website? Many health websites post information collected from other websites or sources. These websites should refer to the original sources of the information and the primary authors. Medical facts and figures posted on websites should have references to the original research articles.

Websites acting as secondary sources can introduce inaccuracies in their coverage of the initial report, even if inadvertent. Popular news media sites may announce preliminary medical findings too premature to be of practical use for you. If you uncover inconsistent statements at different websites acting as secondary sources, then check back to the original source. Furthermore, sites should identify the kind of the evidence on which the materials are based. Traditional medicine and science use stringently controlled experiments and statistical methods to validate its statements. Opinions, anecdotal stories, informal Internet polls, and personal testimonials are unreliable as supporting evidence, if not entirely inaccurate. Websites selling unproven remedies for cancer or promoting fraudulent junk theories about cancer frequently draw on unsubstantiated personal testimonials to persuade their readers.

- How current is the information? Medical information can change frequently; for example, knowledge about GIST has progressed yearly since 2000. A reliable website should be reviewed and updated on a regular basis, with the date of the most recent update clearly indicated (usually at the bottom of the web page).

- What type of personal information does the website collect? Some health-related websites may ask you for personal information in order for you to register or become a member, or you may be charged a fee. Any website asking for personal information should explain clearly what they intend to do with it. Some commercial websites sell compiled user data to other companies. Be certain to understand the site's privacy policy before you submit any personal information.

Search engines help to locate web pages. The search engine scans its database and returns a file with links to websites containing the keyword(s) that you have typed. Unless you provide additional criteria to narrow the search, the list of results can be in the thousands. Search engines allow you to refine your searches so the most relevant websites are at the top of the list. Familiarize yourself with the online tutorials for the search engine's power searching commands. To begin, you must identify the keywords for your topic and determine any synonyms, alternate spellings, or variant word forms for the concepts. Some search strategies include the following:

- Use quotation marks to retrieve phrases where the words appear side by side (e.g., "elevated liver enzymes").
- Combine quoted phrases with Boolean logic to refine the search criteria (AND, OR, and AND NOT). For example, a search of *"GIST" AND "liver enzymes"* would retrieve only those websites containing both of the quoted terms. If you are interested in the effects of cancer on liver enzymes but not in hepatitis, which also elevates liver enzymes, then you could narrow the results by searching for *"cancer" AND "liver enzymes" AND NOT "hepatitis."* In many search engines, the plus (+) and minus symbols (–) are used as alternatives to AND and AND NOT, respectively. There is no space between the plus or minus sign and the keyword.
- Find web pages where the keyword appears in its web address (e.g., *inurl:"GIST"*) or search for certain types of sites containing the keyword (e.g., *site:.gov "GIST"*).
- Use a file type search to retrieve specific types of files containing the keyword (e.g., *filetype:PDF "GIST"*).
- Use a host search to locate keywords within large websites (e.g., *site:www.cancer.gov "surgical resection"*).

100. Where can I learn more information about GIST?

The authors of this book do not necessarily endorse the following additional resources and websites; nevertheless, the resources and websites are intended to provide additional information for managing your illness and making informed decisions about your care. You can find more resources listed in the Resources section of this book.

You can find more resources listed in the index of this book.

- To read basic patient education materials about GIST, see the American Cancer Society (www.cancer.org) and People Living with Cancer (www.plwc.org).
- To search for clinical trials, check National Institutes of Health (www.clinicaltrials.gov) and the NCI PDQ cancer trials (www.cancer.gov/clinicaltrials). EmergingMed is a clinical trial referral service (www.emergingmed.com). No centralized registries for clinical trial offerings exist, and you may need to search several websites to find what you need.
- MedlinePlus from the National Institutes of Health and other trusted sources has extensive information on over 700 diseases and conditions, including an overview of GIST (www.nlm.nih.gov/medlineplus/intestinalcancer.html). MedlinePlus offers many educational resources and information in Spanish.
- Professional societies publish abstracts and online presentations from their annual conferences on their websites, including American Society of Clinical Oncology (www.asco.org) and the Connective Tissue Oncology Society (www.ctos.org). When reading materials written for professionals, keep your focus on understanding the title of the presentation and the one or two sentences that make up the conclusion at the end of the abstract. Use a medical glossary if helpful. Sometimes you can just skip over the complex details within medical abstracts. Try to extract a succinct take-home lesson that you will be able to recite later in plain terms.
- The National Comprehensive Cancer Network (www.nccn.org) has clinical practice guidelines and a directory of physicians and their specialties from 20 National Comprehensive Cancer Network member institutions. GIST is included in the National Compre-

hensive Cancer Network clinical practice guidelines for soft tissue sarcoma.

- PubMed is a free search engine offered by the U.S. National Library of Medicine (www.ncbi.nlm.nih.gov). It searches for published medical and scientific articles from a database of thousands of life science journals. By using the PubMed search engine, you can track the newest as well as the older research articles published about GIST and learn more about emerging cancer drugs. The articles retrieved from a PubMed search for "gastrointestinal stromal tumor" are a good way to become familiar with the names of the doctors and the institutions that actively research this disease.

Resources

Organizations for Patient Support

GIST Support International (www.gistsupport.org)
Life Raft Group (www.liferaftgroup.org)
Das Lebenshaus (www.daslebenshaus.org)
GIST Italian Association (www.gistonline.it)
GIST Support UK (www.gistsupport.co.uk)
Hungarian GIST Group (www.gist.hu)
Japanese Study Group on GIST (www.gist.jp)
Life Raft Group Nederland (www.liferaftgroup.nl)
Polish GIST Society (www.gist.pl)
Swiss GIST Patient's Group (www.gastrointestinale-stromatumoren.com)

GIST Research Fundraising Organizations

GIST Cancer Research Fund (www.gistinfo.org)

Glossary

A

Abdomen: Part of the body between the chest and the pelvis.

Abdominoperineal resection: Removal of the rectum and anus.

Ablation: A surgical procedure that locally destroys a tumor usually by heating or freezing.

Adenocarcinoma: Cancer that begins in cells that line certain internal organs and that has glandular (secretory) properties; most cancers of the stomach and intestines are adenocarcinoma.

Adhesions: Scar tissue that develops after most abdominal operations.

Advance health care directives: Your oral and written instructions about your medical care in the event you become unable to communicate for yourself; includes a health care proxy and a living will.

Advanced GIST: Can refer to a patient who has metastatic disease or unresectable primary GIST.

Anemia: A low level of red blood cells, which carry oxygen in the blood.

Anesthesiologist: A physician who is specially trained to administer anesthesia during surgery.

Anesthetic: A substance that is used to prevent a loss of sensation.

Angina: A disease marked by spasmodic attacks of intense chest pain.

Angiogenesis: The process by which the body forms new small blood vessels called capillaries.

Angiogenesis inhibitors: Substances that stop the formation of new blood vessels.

Anorexia: A loss of appetite.

Anti-angiogenesis drugs: Same as angiogenesis inhibitors.

Antibody: A protein used by pathologists to diagnose the type of a tumor.

Anticipatory grief: Covers the complicated set of emotional reactions and practical adaptations by a family during the lengthy period leading up to the loss of a loved one.

Antisense therapy: Synthetic genetic material that may stop or slow the growth of cancer cells.

Aorta: The large main artery that comes from the left ventricle of the heart that carries oxygenated blood.

Apoptosis: One way in which cells die after being exposed to chemotherapy.

Ascites: The accumulation of fluid in the abdomen.

B

Benign tumor: Although not malignant or cancerous, abnormal tissue that can grow and may even become a larger size. Unlike a cancer, a benign tumor does not invade normal surrounding tissue and does not spread to other organs.

Bereavement: A loss of a loved one by death.

Bile: A brownish, greenish fluid made in the liver and stored in the gallbladder; travels via the bile duct into the second portion of the duodenum. Bile helps in the digestion of fat.

Bilirubin: A red bile substance from the breakdown of red blood cells.

Biological therapy: Treatment modality that uses antibodies, cytokines, and other immune system substances produced in the laboratory to alter the interaction between the body's immune defenses and the cancer cells.

Blood transfusion: The procedure to replace or augment a person's volume of blood.

Botanicals: Any plants (usually herbs or flowers) that are used as medicines.

Bowel obstruction: Condition in which the intestines do not function properly because something is blocking them from emptying.

C

Cachexia: A wasting syndrome in which muscle fibers are broken down for their protein content.

Cancer: A group of diseases in which cells grow abnormally.

Cancer-related fatigue: Different than the tiredness experienced by healthy people after a busy day of ac-

tivities; more severe and not alleviated by more rest and sleep.

Capillaries: Tiny blood vessels that carry oxygen and nutrients, providing cells with the ability to grow.

Cardiologist: A physician specially trained to care for patients with heart problems.

Cardiopulmonary resuscitation: A series of actions and treatments that are used when a patient is no longer breathing or no longer has a pulse.

Cardiovascular: Pertaining to the heart and blood vessels.

Carney's triad: A rare disease in young adults and children in which a GIST occurs in combination with lung and nerve sarcomas. Most patients are female. The GISTs are from the stomach, often multifocal, and lack *KIT* or *PDGFRA* mutations.

Cell: Smallest structural unit of an organism.

Cell death–inducing drugs: Drugs that promote cell death by interfering with proteins that normally act as regulatory counterparts against too many prodeath signals.

Chemotherapy: Treatment with drugs intended to kill cancer cells.

Chromosome: Thread-like strand of DNA and other proteins that carry the genes and functions to provide hereditary information.

Chronic myeloid leukemia: A slowly progressing disease in which too many white blood cells are made in the bone marrow.

Clinical trials: A research study that allows physicians to answer specific medical questions, usually about treatments.

Colon: Also called the large intestine; reabsorbs water and salts from the intestinal contents.

Colonoscopy: Also called a lower endoscopy; can detect abnormalities of the rectum and large colon.

Colorectal surgeon: A surgeon who specializes in colon surgery.

Colostomy: The surgical construction of an artificial opening into the colon that allows fecal material to empty into a bag.

Complementary and alternative medicine: Approaches to health care that are outside the realm of conventional medicine; can be used either with conventional medicine (complementary) or in place of it (alternative).

Complete blood count: A blood test that measures the number, type, and/or size of red blood cells, white blood cells, and platelets.

Compliance: Act of following a treatment plan consistently and correctly.

Congestive heart failure: A condition in which the heart does not pump effectively.

Contrast: A special type of dye that is given orally, intravenously, or rectally; the dye makes the images show up better on various radiographic studies or MRIs.

Cryotherapy: Technique of inserting a metal probe into the tumor and exposing it to extreme cold.

CT scan: Also called a CAT scan (computed tomography); a series of X-rays that are reconstructed to provide cross-sectional images of your body.

Cytokines: Proteins that are secreted by tumors and increase body's need for energy; weaken muscles and cause low-grade fevers.

D

Depression: A disorder characterized by persistent sadness, sense of loss or hopelessness, sleeplessness, and/or loss of appetite or energy,

Dietary supplements: Any substance added to the diet, such as vitamins, minerals, or herbs, in addition to what the body already takes in.

Disease progression: Cancer that continues to grow or spread.

Diuretic: A medication used to treat the accumulation of too much fluid in the body (edema); assists in the discharge of the fluid through urine.

DNA: Deoxyribonucleic acid. A nucleic acid that carries the genetic information in the cell. DNA consists of two long chains of nucleotides twisted into a double helix to form chromosomes.

DNA base sequence: The linear order of the four types of nucleotide bases in a DNA molecule; determines structure of proteins encoded by the DNA.

Do-Not-Intubate (DNI) order: An advance directive that says that the patient should not be intubated (with a plastic mouthpiece and tube) in the event that the patient stops breathing or no longer has a pulse.

Do-Not-Resuscitate (DNR) order: An advance directive that says that CPR should not be performed in the event the patient stops breathing or no longer has a pulse.

Dumping syndrome: A potential complication of removing the stomach in which diarrhea and skin flushing are present after eating a meal; generally treated with diet modification.

Duodenum: First 12 inches of the small intestine.

Durable power of attorney for health care: The legal document that authorizes a person to serve as a patient's health care proxy.

E

Echocardiogram: An ultrasound of the heart that examines its structure and function.

Edema: Excessive accumulation of fluid.

Electrocardiogram: ECG or EKG, tracing of the electrical impulses of the heart.

Embolization: Treatment to block the flow of blood to a tumor.

Endoscope: An instrument used to examine the inside of organs, most usually the esophagus, stomach, and duodenum.

Endoscopic ultrasound (EUS): Ultrasound (using sound waves) test performed during endoscopy.

Endoscopy: Refers to examination of any body part with an instrument composed of light and tubing; most commonly refers to examining the upper gastrointestinal tract into part of the small intestine.

Enteral nutrition: Nutrition provided though a tube inserted into the stomach or intestine.

Enzyme: Any of numerous complex proteins that are produced by living cells and assist specific biochemical reactions at body temperatures.

Epithelial cells: One of many kinds of cells that form the epithelium and absorb nutrients.

Epithelioid: Cell morphology (shape and appearance) that looks round or polygonal.

Epoetin alpha: A drug used to treat some forms of anemia; a man-made preparation of the human growth factor erythropoietin that stimulates production of red blood cells.

Esophagus: Primarily a passageway that pushes and moves food to the stomach.

Exon: A specific portion of a gene that codes for part of a protein.

F

Fine-needle aspiration: A procedure performed by using a thin needle to obtain a few cells for examination.

Foley catheter: A narrow tube placed in the bladder so that the amount of urine can be closely monitored.

G

Gastrectomy: Removal of the stomach.

Gastritis: Inflammation of the stomach.

Gastroenterologist: A physician specially trained in the field of diseases related to the gastrointestinal tract and organs in the abdomen.

Gastrointestinal stromal tumor: A type of cancer classified as a sarcoma. GIST is thought to originate from a special type of nerve cell in the gastrointestinal tract called the intestinal cell of Cajal.

Gastrointestinal tract: The mouth, esophagus, stomach, small intestine, large intestine, rectum, and anus.

Gene: Hereditary unit on a chromosome.

Gene therapy: Treatment that attempts to correct errors in cells that have missing genes or too many other genes.

Growth factors: Proteins in the body that activate cells to grow.

Guaiac test: A lab test using a small amount of stool placed on a special card to look for blood; this investigation may be performed during routine physical examination, or it may be prompted by a low blood count on routine blood tests.

H

Health care proxy: A person appointed to make a patient's medical decisions if the patient is unable to do so.

Hematoma: A break in a blood vessel causing swelling.

Hemoglobin: The oxygen-carrying component of red blood cells.

Hepatic artery: An artery that carries blood to the liver.

Hepatic artery embolization: The injection of particles into the hepatic artery in order to destroy a GIST that has spread to the liver.

Hepatobiliary surgeon: A surgeon who operates on the liver and pancreas.

Hiatal hernia: Slippage of part of the stomach from the abdomen to the chest.

Hospice: A philosophy about end-of-life care, not a specific place of care; appropriate when a patient can no longer benefit from cancer treatments and has a limited life expectancy, generally 6 months or less. The principal aim is to maintain quality of life during the last stages of incurable disease.

Hypertension: Abnormally high arterial blood pressure that is usually indicated by an adult systolic blood pressure of 140 mm Hg or greater or a diastolic blood pressure of 90 mm Hg or greater.

Hypothyroidism: Deficient activity of the thyroid gland.

I

Imatinib: A targeted cancer therapy called a kinase inhibitor; used in the treatment of a type of leukemia and in GISTs.

Immune system: The integrated body system that protects the body from infections and diseases.

Immunohistochemistry: Microscopic examination of cells by staining them with antibodies.

Incidentally: Detected by accident.

Incisions: Surgical cuts in the skin.

Informed consent: When a patient agrees to a certain procedure or treatment by signing an agreement that says the patient understands the procedure or treatment, the risks, and benefits and that the rights and safety of the patient have been discussed.

Interventional radiologist: A radiologist who uses image guidance to gain access to vessels and organs in order to treat conditions under the skin; uses catheters, balloons, and stents.

Intravenous: Through the vein.

Iron-deficiency anemia: Anemia caused by lack of iron in the diet or from chronic bleeding.

J

Jaundice: Yellowish discoloration of the skin, whites of the eyes, and mucous membranes from the accumulation of bile salts; symptom of liver diseases.

L

Laparoscopy: Performed under general anesthesia; a few small incisions (less than an inch) are made in order to insert a telescope and some instruments in order to inspect the organs of the abdomen and/or pelvis.

Laparotomy: An incision into the abdomen.

Leiomyosarcomas: Another type of sarcoma that can arise from the gastrointestinal tract; less common than GISTs; smooth muscle sarcomas.

Liver: Organ in the right upper abdomen that secretes bile and assists in the metabolism of many substances, including proteins and many medications; common site of metastases.

Liver toxicity: Liver that retains toxins from metabolizing drugs; can be a life-threatening condition.

Living will: Specific instructions regarding measures that would prolong life, outlining the medical interventions to be performed or withheld, including life-sustaining procedures or artificial life support in the event the patient can no longer communicate.

Lower endoscopy: See colonoscopy.

Lung chondroma: A benign growth of cartilage-producing cells that should not ordinarily be in the lungs.

Lymph nodes: The small roundish bodies located in chains around the body that act like filters for certain substances in the blood and tissue; store certain type of white cells; common site of metastases of many cancers, but not GISTs.

Lymphoma: Cancer that arises from cells in the immune system.

M

Malnutrition: State of poor nutrition as a result of faulty digestion or poorly balanced diet.

Mass: Often used interchangeably with tumor; sometimes the group of cells that make up a mass have an unknown origin.

Medical oncologist: A cancer specialist that specializes in the use of chemotherapy, biologic, and other nonsurgical treatments of cancer.

Megadosing: Excessive doses of vitamins and supplements beyond the recommended daily amount thought to improve health.

Melanoma: A form of skin cancer that can begin as a mole or a darkly pigmented area on the skin.

Melena: Dark, tarry stools.

Mental imagery: Technique used to visualize pleasant scenes in the mind; often used as a stress management tool.

Mesentery: Fatty tissue around the intestines.

Metabolic panel: Tests of certain substances in blood that determine whether the kidneys and liver are functioning normally; tests include but are not limited to the following: blood urea nitrogen, creatinine, total protein, albumin, bilirubin, AST, ALT, and alkaline phosphatase.

Metabolism: The breaking down of substances in the body to generate energy.

Metastasis: The process of spreading cancer cells from the primary site to somewhere else in the body.

Metastatic GIST: A GIST that has spread to another organ or site from the primary tumor, which may or may not have been already removed.

Mind–body connection: Belief that the mind can help to heal the body.

Mitotic rate: The rate at which cells divide.

Molecular tests: Tests of molecules essential to life such as nucleic acids and their role in genetic information.

Molecular-targeted drugs or molecularly targeted therapies: Drugs that work precisely against particular abnormal molecules within a type of cancer.

MRI: Also called MR (magnetic resonance imaging) provides cross-sectional images of the body; uses a magnetic field, instead of radiation, to generate images.

Multikinase inhibitors: Drugs that block multiple kinases (proteins) within a cell.

Mutation: Any change in the base sequence of the DNA of a cell.

Mutational status: The type of mutation within a tumor.

N

Narcotic: A potent drug derived from opium or opium-like compounds given to relieve pain; associated with significant effects on mood and behavior with the potential for dependence and tolerance.

Needle biopsy: The insertion of a needle into a tumor to obtain a few of its cells for the purposes of examining the cells.

Negative margin of resection: No cancer cells are found in the edge of the surrounding tissue that's removed along with the tumor.

Neoadjuvant therapy: Chemotherapy or targeted therapy administered before surgery; goal is to shrink the tumor to make the tumor completely removable, reduce the risk of the operation, or decrease the amount of normal tissue that needs to be sacrificed.

Neuroendocrine: Relating to the hormones of endocrine glands.

Neurofibromatosis: A genetic disease characterized by pigmented skin lesions, sometimes tumors that cause deformity, and predisposition to certain types of cancer.

Neutropenia: Low level of white blood cells.

Neutrophil: White blood cell that destroys microorganisms and fights infection.

Neutrophilia: An increase in the number of neutrophils in the blood.

O

Omentum: Fatty areas around the stomach.

Over-the-counter medication: Describes medications, herbs, or supplements that can be purchased without a prescription.

P

Pancreas: A large lobulated gland located behind the stomach and closely associated with the duodenum. It makes enzymes to digest food and regulates your blood sugar level.

Pancreaticoduodenectomy: See Whipple procedure.

Paraganglioma: A type of nerve sarcoma.

Parenteral nutrition: Nutrition infused into the bloodstream.

Pathologist: A physician trained in the structural and functional changes that result from disease processes; examines tissues for evidence of disease.

Percutaneous: Through the skin.

Peritoneum: A thin layer of tissue that covers abdominal organs.

Persistency: Taking drug on an uninterrupted basis for the entire duration of the therapy.

PET flare: A sign on the PET scan that the tumors again have high metabolic activity.

PET scan: Positron emission tomography, a nuclear medicine test; a special type of sugar is injected into a vein, and then images are taken that show how the sugar is taken up by different parts of your body.

Phase I: The study that primarily establishes the safety of a newly discovered drug or a combination of drugs, while studying the efficacy in many diseases.

Phase II: The study that primarily evaluates the efficacy of a drug or a combination of drugs in a specific disease.

Phase III: The study that compares the experimental drug or drugs with the standard care of this disease or a placebo.

Placebo: An inactive substance that contains no medication or active ingredient to be given to participants in a clinical trial to determine the effectiveness of a particular medication or substance given to other participants.

Platelets: Found in blood; assists in clotting of blood.

Pleural effusion: Fluid in the lungs.

Pneumonia: A disease of the lungs that is usually caused by infection. It is accompanied by fever, chills, cough, and difficulty in breathing.

Portal vein: A vein entering the liver.

Preoperative: Before surgery.

Primary localized GIST: The GIST tumor is found in only one place and shows no evidence of spread to other sites.

Primary mutation: The mutations that exists in a tumor prior to any therapy.

Primary site: The initial site of origin of a cancer.

Prognosis: Prediction of the course of an illness.

Protein: Large molecules made of amino acids. Proteins participate in all essential processes in a cell, and form a body's major structures.

Protocol: The ultimate reference for clinical trials that describes all the rules and conditions that govern the trial; ensures the quality of the trial and thus its reproducibility, as well as the safety and protection of the patients in the trial.

Pseudoaneurysm: An abnormal dilation of the arterial wall at a previous site of catheter entry.

Psychiatrist: A physician specially trained in the diagnosis and treatment of mental health disorders.

Pulmonary embolus: A blood clot that lodges in the lung.

Q

Quackery: Refers to the promotion of methods or products that are known to be false or unproven.

R

Radiation oncologist: A doctor who specializes in using radiation to treat cancer.

Radiation therapy: A treatment modality that depends on the high energy of certain electromagnetic waves controlled and directed toward a cancer; the two main types of radiation waves are X-rays and gamma rays.

Radiofrequency ablation: Technique of inserting a metal probe into the tumor and exposing it to extreme heat.

Radiologist: A physician specially trained in the interpretation of imaging studies; a diagnostic radiologist reads conventional X-rays, CT scans, and MRIs; a nuclear medicine radiologist reads PET scans, and an interventional radiologist performs procedures.

Receptor tyrosine kinases: A group of proteins on the cell surface involved in signal transduction.

Rectum: Approximately 12 cm long and functions as a storage tank of fecal material at the end of the large intestine; emptied on defecation.

Recurrent cancer: Cancer that comes back in a patient who appeared cancer free for a time.

Red blood cells: A blood cell that contains hemoglobin and transports oxygen and carbon dioxide to and from tissues.

Resection: Surgical removal of an organ or other body structure.

Resistance: Lack of response of a cancer to treatment.

S

Saliva: A substance in the mouth that provides lubrication and initiates digestion.

Sarcomas: Cancers that arise from components of nerve tissue, connective tissue, or muscle and therefore can occur anywhere in the body.

Secondary mutation: A second distinct mutation in the *KIT* or *PDGFRA* genes arising in addition to the primary mutation; a major cause of acquired resistance to drug therapy.

Signal transduction: The internal cellular processes that relay chemical messages from the cell surface into its nucleus (where genes are located) or into other cellular compartments.

Signal transduction inhibitors: Small molecules which interfere with cell surface receptors that relay growth signals from the environment into the cell; may also inhibit proteins within cells that speed up the chemical reactions for growth.

Spindle: Cell morphology (shape and appearance) that looks long and thin.

Spleen: A highly vascular abdominal organ that filters the blood and contributes to the immune system.

Stress test: A test that measures heart function during strenuous exercise or after medication is given.

Subtypes: Different types stemming from the main type.

Sunitinib: A kinase inhibitor and anti-angiogenesis drug used to treat advanced kidney cancer and metastatic GISTs.

Surgical margins: The amount of normal tissue that the surgeon removed around the tumor.

Surgical oncologist: A surgeon who specializes in the surgical treatment of cancer.

T

Targeted cancer therapy: Treatments of drugs or other substances intended to attack cancer cells and not normal cells.

Terminal: Disease that cannot be cured and will cause death.

Toxicities: Undesirable side effects from medications.

Tru-cut biopsy: A procedure performed through the skin to obtain a larger sample of tissue for diagnosis; performed under CT or ultrasound guidance.

Tumor ablation: The destruction of a tumor without actually removing it.

Tumor progression: Enlarging or spreading of the tumor.

Tyrosine kinase inhibitors: A group of drugs that block the function of certain proteins responsible for stimulating the growth of cancer cells.

U

Upper endoscopy: Performed by inserting a scope into your mouth in order to examine the esophagus, stomach, and duodenum.

Urogenital: Related to the urinary excretion or reproductive systems.

V

Vascular endothelial growth factor (VEGF): A substance that stimulates the growth of the endothelial cells required to form capillaries.

Vitamin B$_{12}$: A vitamin needed to treat pernicious anemia, a form of anemia resulting from stomach disturbances that prevent the absorption of B$_{12}$.

W

Whipple procedure: Operation in which part of the pancreas, a small piece of intestine, possibly part of the stomach, part of the bile duct, and gallbladder are removed. Also called pancreaticoduodenectomy.

White blood cells: Blood cells that protect the body from infection or disease.

INDEX

Index